FAST FACTS FOR THE ER NURSE

About the Author

Jennifer R. Buettner, RN, CEN, is currently a full-time Registered Nurse at Emory University Hospital Midtown's emergency room in Atlanta, GA. She has ten years of ER experience and three years of experience precepting new graduate nurses and new employees in the ER. She is Certified in Emergency Nursing (CEN), ACLS, PALS, TNCC, and as Nurse Preceptor (Rockdale Medical Center/2005) and is a member of the Emergency Nurses' Association. Jennifer won the Faculty Award for the graduate who "has achieved excellence in both the academic and clinical settings and who best exemplifies the total integration of program philosophy to professional performance" (3/1999). She has developed an ER Orientation Packet and Education Course for two local hospitals. Her book derives from her inability to find an orientation manual that was sized and priced reasonably enough for hospital ERs to purchase in sufficient quantities to provide to all preceptors and new ER nurses.

FAST FACTS FOR THE ER NURSE

Emergency Room Orientation in a Nutshell

Jennifer R. Buettner, RN, CEN

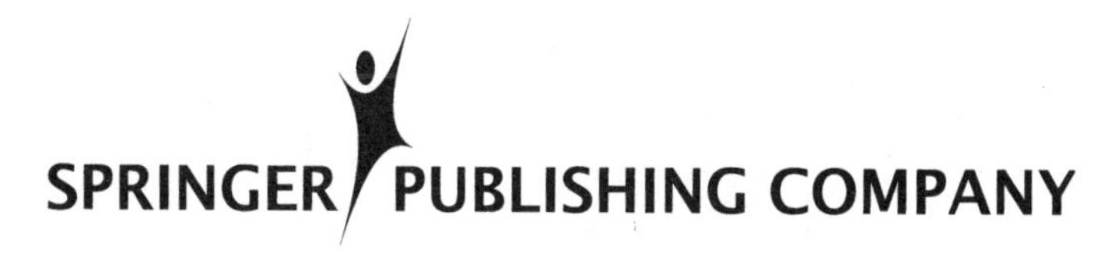

New York

Springer Publishing Company, LLC
11 West 42nd Street
New York, NY 10036
www.springerpub.com

Acquisitions Editor: Margaret Zuccarini
Production Editor: Barbara A. Chernow
Cover design: David Levy
Composition: Agnew's, Inc.

Ebook ISBN: 978-0-8261-0522-6

12/ 6

The author and the publisher of this Work have made every effort to use sources believed to be reliable to provide information that is accurate and compatible with the standards generally accepted at the time of publication. Because medical science is continually advancing, our knowledge base continues to expand. Therefore, as new information becomes available, changes in procedures become necessary. We recommend that the reader always consult current research and specific institutional policies before performing any clinical procedure. The author and publisher shall not be liable for any special, consequential, or exemplary damages resulting, in whole or in part, from the readers' use of, or reliance on, the information contained in this book. The publisher has no responsibility for the persistence or accuracy of URLs for external or third-party Internet Web sites referred to in this publication and does not guarantee that any content on such Web sites is, or will remain, accurate or appropriate.

Library of Congress Cataloging-in-Publication Data

Buettner, Jennifer R.
Fast facts for the ER nurse : emergency room orientation in a nutshell / by Jennifer R. Buettner.
p. ; cm.
Includes bibliographical references and index.
ISBN 978-0-8261-0521-9
1. Emergency nursing—Handbooks, manuals, etc. I. Title.
[DNLM: 1. Emergencies—nursing—Handbooks. 2. Emergency Nursing—methods—Handbooks. WY 49 B928f 2009]
RT120.E4B84 2009
616.02'5—dc22

2009015441

Printed in the United States of America by Hamilton Printing

To emergency nurses everywhere. May God bless your hands as you touch so many patients' lives.

Contents

Appendices

Preface

This is a book designed for *real* emergency room nurses by a *real* emergency room nurse. This quick reference is intended to aid your day-to-day emergency room orientation process with your preceptor. This book will help guide you through the most common illnesses seen in the emergency department. This book does not cover basic anatomy and physiology, advanced cardiovascular life support, pediatric advanced life support, or the trauma nurse core course. The information in this book is compiled from basic emergency room knowledge and the sources used are believed to be reliable. There are several points to take into consideration in referencing this book. First, all listed interventions that go beyond the Scope of Nursing Practice should be followed as ordered by the Emergency Room (ER) Provider. Secondly, the term Provider in this book could be a physician (MD or DO), a nurse practitioner (NP), or a physician assistant (PA), who is qualified to provide such ER patient care. In most cases, interventions that go beyond the usual Scope of Nursing Practice have been introduced using "Anticipate an order to:" followed by a list of possible Provider orders. As always, it is the responsibility of the nurse to check any noted medication dosages or treatments to ensure that all are current, recommended, and accepted practice. After reading this book, you will become the jack of all illnesses, master of none. So, put on your running shoes, keep a stash of chocolates, and when all else fails, practice unreasonable happiness. One thing is for sure; just when you think you have seen it all, your next patient will come in.

Each chapter includes a brief introduction; an outline of materials, equipment, and drugs with which you should become familiar; a list of diagnoses that includes definitions, causes, signs and symptoms, and interventions; and a feature entitled "Fast facts in a nutshell" that provides quick summaries of important points or questions and answers for your review. The end of the book includes appendices, including a list of abbreviations, Common Lab Values, and frequently used ER medications, that should become second nature to all emergency room personnel.

There are two ways to use this book. You can review the book cover to cover, or you can use the skills check-off sheets in Appendix E and review the appropriate chapters.

Jennifer R. Buettner, RN, CEN

Acknowledgments

I could not do what I do without the support of my family, but the base of my emergency nursing foundation was built by my first preceptor, Linda Whitt, RN. Thank you for sharing your wealth of knowledge and setting a prime example of a truly caring and compassionate nurse. I can't forget my second preceptor, Walter McCracken, RN, whose pearls of wisdom can be found in no book. I would also like to thank all my coworkers, who have inspired and molded me into the nurse I am today.

I would like to acknowledge the work of the following individuals for reviewing the manuscript for accuracy: Heather Hall, MD, Nichole Lunsford, RN, Cyndi Griffith, RN, Laura Phillips, RN, and Teresa M. Campo, DNP, RN, NP-C.

Last, but not least, I would like to thank the nurse and friend who inspired me to write this book, Nichole Lunsford, RN. Above all, my faith has sustained me through all my endeavors; I would like to thank God for all of His gifts and blessings.

FAST FACTS FOR THE ER NURSE

Chapter 1

Tips on Surviving ER Nursing

INTRODUCTION

Even if you love working in the emergency room, it can be tough at times. The emergency room is particularly stressful because you care for a broad spectrum of patients in a fast-paced, critical environment. So, not only do you need to be extremely knowledgeable, you also need to be organized, calm, and fast on your feet. Everyone knows that the nurses are the very heart of the emergency room. Your patients rely on you. But ***to take care of others, you first need to take care of yourself*** *physically, mentally, and spiritually. This chapter includes a checklist of stress symptoms and a list of simple methods for coping with those pressures.*

During this part of your orientation, you will learn:

1. How to recognize the symptoms of stress on the job.
2. Basic techniques you can use on the job to alleviate that stress.

SYMPTOMS OF STRESS

It is true that ER nurses are sometimes referred to as "adrenaline junkies." However, one can not function on adrenaline alone. Severe stress and anxiety on the job is harmful to you and your patients. So learn to recognize the signs and symptoms: severe muscle tension, fatigue, irritability, flight or fight response, tachycardia, tachypnea, weakness, sweating, feeling helpless, angry, tearful, urinary urgency, diarrhea, dry mouth, insomnia, difficulty in problem solving, feeling overwhelmed, and decreased appetite.

> **Fast facts in a nutshell**
>
> To take care of others, you first need to take care of yourself.

TECHNIQUES FOR RELIEVING STRESS

1. Take a moment, close your eyes and take some deep cleansing breaths. Breathe in through your nose as you count to five. Then exhale slowly through your mouth as you count to five, and that's it. Breathing exercises increase oxygen to your brain and are a fast, simple way to relieve stress anytime, anywhere.
2. Stay hydrated. Keep a water bottle with you at work. Staying hydrated is an easy way to stay healthy.

3. Focus on the positives. When you have a complaint, spend your energy finding a solution rather than complaining. You need all the energy you can get, so use it to resolve stressful problems.
4. Leave your work at work, and your home life at home. Divide and conquer your stressors.
5. Listen to upbeat energizing music on the way to work so that the melody will repeat itself in your head all day. "Whistle while you work." Singing or humming is a good way to relieve stress.
6. Keep a stash of *dark* chocolates: they are actually a source of energy and antioxidants. Dark chocolate not only boosts your immune system, it seems to make people happy. It works well on any grumpy coworkers too, so don't forget to share.
7. Introduce yourself to patients when you enter a room. Keeping the patient informed of who you are and what you are going to be doing relieves their stress.
8. Wear a well-made and comfortable pair of shoes. Eight to 12 hours of painful swollen feet will only add to your stress.
9. Recognize that it is perfectly normal to feel anxious during a code (e.g., cardiac/pulmonary arrest). Only time and training will help you cope with the anxiety felt when performing advanced cardiovascular life supportive treatments.
10. Do not think or act as if you know it all. Medicine is constantly changing. No matter how much emergency room experience you have, you can still learn something new every day.

11. Keep the following in your pocket every day: trauma shears, hemostats, tape, pen, calculator (with list of emergency room intravenous drips and doses taped to back) and this book. Being prepared will reduce stress and anxiety.
12. Invest in a good pair of support hose and do leg exercises. Most nurses develop varicose veins. It is hard to take good care of your patients when your legs ache and have poor circulation.
13. Ask or look up any medications about which you are unsure. There are numerous medication routes and doses to memorize. Looking them up or asking will help you learn them and keep your patients safe and free of medication errors.
14. Keep your uniforms clean, to save you the hassle from having to buy new scrubs frequently. Wash out betadine or benzoic stains on your scrubs with rubbing alcohol. Pour hydrogen peroxide on any blood spots on your uniform, and let foam for a minute. Then wash with soap and water.
15. Have a sense of humor even if it seems unreasonable. You won't survive without one. Laughter is often the best medicine.
17. Avoid gossip. If you don't have anything nice to say, don't say anything at all. We are all on the same team. We need to build each other up, not tear each other down.
18. Increase your emergency room knowledge. Join the Emergency Nurses Association, sign up for emergency room-related courses, and study from a CEN review book. Increasing your knowledge base is key for better patient care.

19. Maintain liability insurance on yourself. It is inexpensive and almost everyone that works in the emergency room, at some point, gets sued. Liability insurance is a simple way to protect yourself.
20. Document, Document, Document! How was the patient when he/she came in? Stable? Pink? Warm? Dry? Any distress? Chart on your nonurgent patient at least every hour; on a critical patient, every 5 to 10 minutes. Chart when you assumed care of the patient. Document how they were when they left the emergency room (e.g., ambulatory, stable, no acute distress) and reassess ABCs.

Fast facts in a nutshell

- Maintain liability insurance on yourself.
- Document, Document, Document!

Fast facts in a nutshell: summary

Emergency nursing is not for everyone. It can be indescribably hard at times. But if you practice these simple stress-relieving techniques you will be able to survive whatever the emergency room throws at you. If you can make it through the tough times, you'll survive long enough to find out just how rewarding emergency room nursing can be. After all, that is why you chose this profession.

Chapter 2

Acid-Base Imbalances

INTRODUCTION

The body requires a delicate balance of acids and bases to maintain natural homeostasis. *Many life-threatening illnesses affect the acid-base balance. Therefore, recognizing any acid-base imbalance is crucial to saving someone's life. As a nurse in the emergency room, you will come across acid-base imbalances daily. Many new and experienced nurses find acid-base balance difficult to understand. After reviewing this chapter and learning the three simple steps provided, you will find it much easier to remember how to interpret test results.* ***Understanding the pathophysiology and reviewing many laboratory results are key to better understanding acid-base imbalances.***

During this part of your orientation, locate and become familiar with:

1. Arterial blood gas procedures and results.
2. Diabetic ketoacidosis protocols.

3. Intubation equipment.
4. Medications: insulin, sodium bicarbonate, potassium, and dextrose.

PATHOPHYSIOLOGY

Acid-base balance is controlled by two organ systems.

Respiratory System

You breathe in oxygen (O_2) and breathe out carbon dioxide (CO_2). In the bloodstream CO_2 mixes with H_2O (water) to make (H_2CO_3) carbonic acid.

Renal System

H_2CO_3 dissociates into a base (HCO_3^-) and an acid (H^+) that are excreted by the kidneys.

Recognizing an Imbalance

An easy way to remember if your patient has a respiratory or metabolic imbalance shown in Table 2.1 is this simple mnemonic.

*Mnemonic for pH/bicarbonate directions in acidosis versus alkalosis, remember **ROME***

***R**espiratory is **O**pposite, **M**etabolic is **E**qual*

TABLE 2.1 Determining Acid-Base Imbalances

Respiratory Acidosis	pH↓	$PaCO_2$↑	HCO_3^- Normal
Respiratory Alkalosis	pH↑	$PaCO_2$↓	HCO_3^- Normal
Metabolic Acidosis	pH↓	$PaCO_2$ Normal	HCO_3^-↓
Metabolic Alkalosis	pH↑	$PaCO_2$ Normal	HCO_3^-↑

Normal pH = 7.35–7.45, Normal $PaCO_2$ = 35–45, Normal HCO_3^- = 22–26

The arrows in Table 2.1 for respiratory pH and $PaCO_2$ are in opposite directions from each other, and the arrows for metabolic pH and bicarbonate are equal or in the same direction.

Fast facts in a nutshell

1. Acid-base balance is controlled by the respiratory and renal systems.

DIAGNOSES

Every acid-base imbalance is described using three words, such as: Uncompensated Respiratory Acidosis. To determine which imbalance your patient has, follow these three simple steps. Table 2.1 provides a visual guide of these steps.

1. Look at the pH. If it is normal (7.35–7.45) it is **compensated.** If it is out of range it is **uncompensated.**
2. A pH below 7.35 is **acidosis.** A pH above 7.45 is **alkalosis.**
3. Look at $PaCO_2$ and HCO_3^-. Abnormal $PaCO_2$ = **respiratory.** Abnormal HCO_3^- = **metabolic.** If both are abnormal it is both **respiratory and metabolic.**

Respiratory Acidosis

In respiratory acidosis, pH is less than 7.35 because of inadequate ventilations. Poor ventilation causes one to retain CO_2. Poor ventilations also lead to poor oxygenation. That means oxygen cannot get in, and CO_2 cannot get out. CO_2 builds up, mixes with H_2O, resulting in carbonic acid (H_2CO_3). Bicarbonate (HCO_3^-) is normal. This patient is at risk for hypoxia.

1. *Causes:* upper airway obstruction; pulmonary edema; hypoventilation; head trauma; chest trauma; pneumonia; chronic obstructive pulmonary disease (COPD); narcotic overdose; and muscle weakness.
2. *Signs and symptoms:* tachycardia; headache; confusion; weakness; coma; cyanosis; bradypnea; paralysis; respiratory arrest.
3. *Interventions:* administer oxygen; nebulized breathing treatments; treat underlying condition; prepare for intubation; provide mechanical ventilation; measure pulse oxygen; monitor cardiac rhythm; and obtain an intravenous access.

Fast facts in a nutshell

Question: What supplies are needed to intubate a patient?
Answer: *High flow oxygen, suction, ambu bag, appropriate size endotracheal tube, 10-ml syringe of air, stylett, appropriate blades (Miller/Abbott) with working handle, CO_2 detector, tape or endotracheal tube securing device, and stethoscope to check placement.*

*Notes:*____________________________________

____

____

Respiratory Alkalosis

In respiratory alkalosis, pH is greater than 7.45. When a person hyperventilates, he/she blows off all of his/her CO_2. There is no CO_2 left to mix with H_2O to make carbonic acid (H_2CO_3). No acid = alkalosis. HCO_3^- is normal.

1. *Causes:* hyperventilation; pain; anxiety; pulmonary embolus; hypoxia; high altitude; drug toxicity (early salicylate adult overdose); third trimester pregnancy; and fever.
2. *Signs and symptoms:* tetany or seizures from hypocalcemia; tingling of extremities; dizziness; altered mental status;

anxiety; paresthesias; palpitations; tachycardia; and hyperventilation.

3. *Interventions:* encourage slow deep breathing; correct underlying condition; provide fluids intravenously; and correct hyperventilation with nonrebreather mask *without* oxygen.
   - Hyperventilation treatment: put oxygen nonrebreather mask over the patient's face and leave turned off. (It works like a paper bag.)

Notes: ______________________________________

____

____

Metabolic Acidosis

In metabolic acidosis, pH is less than 7.35 due to a decrease in (bicarbonate) HCO_3^- or increase in H^+ ion. $PaCO_2$ is normal.

1. *Causes:* diabetic ketoacidosis; renal disease; starvation; shock or sepsis; and loss of bicarbonate in severe diarrhea.
2. *Signs and symptoms:* altered mental state; hypotension; abdominal pain; nausea, vomiting, and diarrhea; Kussmaul respirations; hyperventilation as a compensatory mechanism; hyperkalemia; flushed, warm skin; bradycardia; and muscle weakness.
3. *Interventions:* provide fluids intravenously (lactated Ringer's); treatment may include intravenous sodium bicarbon-

ate, intravenous dextrose and intravenous regular insulin (to put potassium back in cells); assist ventilations; monitor cardiac rhythm; and perform basic metabolic panel.

Diabetic Ketoacidosis (DKA)

Diabetic keoacidosis is a state of metabolic acidosis that is the result of elevated blood sugar (greater than 300). When the blood sugar is this high, the body does not have sufficient insulin to break down sugar for energy. To compensate, the body breaks down fat, thereby releasing toxic ketone acids.

1. *Causes:* uncontrolled blood sugar in diabetes mellitus.
2. *Signs and symptoms:* dry, flushed skin; serum glucose level greater than 300; nausea and vomiting; increased thirst; urinary frequency; weakness; Kussmaul breathing; ketones in urine; change in level of consciousness; and coma.
3. *Interventions:* obtain and monitor blood sugar every hour; monitor acetone level; check arterial blood gases; perform basic metabolic panel and urinalysis; monitor cardiac rhythm; administer 2 liters of oxygen by nasal cannula; administer intravenous normal saline bolus; medicate for nausea and vomiting; and give insulin (first, 5 to 10 units of regular intravenous push, and then 0.1 units per kilogram per hour by intravenous fusion on a pump). Once the patient's blood sugar is below 250, change from intravenous to subcutaneous insulin per the provider's order. Then also change the intravenous solution from normal saline to 5% Dextrose 0.45% normal saline (D_5 ½NS)

at a rate of 150 to 200 ml per hour per the provider's order. Prepare for possible intensive care unit admission.

- Once you replace fluids be prepared for urinary frequency. Provide urinals, Foley cath, or bedpans. Collect urinalysis and monitor intake and output.

Notes: ______________________________

____

____

Metabolic Alkalosis

In metabolic alkalosis, the pH is greater than 7.45 due to elevated HCO_3^- or decreased H^+. $PaCO_2$ is normal.

1. *Causes:* loss of stomach acid associated with vomiting; ingesting too many alkali substances (antacids, milk of magnesia, or baking soda); diuretics; hypokalemia; and Cushing's syndrome.
2. *Signs and symptoms:* hypocalcemia (tetany, twitching, shaking, seizures); confusion; nausea, vomiting, and diarrhea; coma; decreased ST segment; bradypnea; hypokalemia (muscle weakness); and polyuria.
3. *Interventions:* anticipate orders to: prevent vomiting with antiemetics, avoid gastric suctioning, administer normal saline intravenously, perform basic metabolic panel (BMP), provide potassium supplements for hypokalemia, monitor cardiac performance and respirations.

Fast facts in a nutshell

Question: Before your patient has an arterial blood gas drawn, what test should be performed?
Answer: *Allen's Test.*

Question: A 29-year-old diabetic female arrives who has dried skin, is flushed, is hot, and has Kussmaul's respirations. What is the underlying illness?
Answer: *Diabetic ketoacidosis—check her blood sugar.*

Question: Your patient is diagnosed with ketoacidosis. What should initial management include?
Answer: *Administering regular insulin intravenously or subcutaneously, followed by an insulin intravenous drip.*

Question: How often should you check blood sugars on a patient receiving an insulin intravenous drip?
Answer: *Every hour.*

Notes: ______________________________

____

____

Fast facts in a nutshell: summary

Although acid-base imbalances can be challenging to understand, they are critical to maintaining natural homeostasis. An emergency room nurse comes across acid-base imbalances on a daily basis. Learn the steps provided in this chapter so you will be able to accurately interpret test results.

Chapter 3

Cardiovascular Emergencies

INTRODUCTION

In the emergency room, cardiovascular diseases are an everyday life-threatening occurrence. However, ***with proper assessment and fast treatment, cardiac diseases are resolved every day in emergency rooms*** *across the country. After studying this chapter, you will have a basic understanding of cardiovascular assessments and treatments. This chapter does not replace electrocardiogram courses or the advanced cardiovascular life support certification required to work in the emergency room.* ***Many nurses find keeping an advanced cardiovascular life support handbook for study is very helpful.***

During this part of your orientation, locate and become familiar with:

1. Electrocardiograms and supplies.
2. Advanced cardiovascular life support and electrocardiogram courses available to you.

3. Cardiac monitors, defibrillators, and pacers.
4. Crash carts.
5. Drugs to know: ASA, morphine, nitroglycerin, atropine, adenosine, digoxin, furosemide, calcium channel blockers, beta blockers, amiodarone, lidocaine, epinephrine, heparin, warfarin, dopamine, and norepinephrine.

DIAGNOSES

Congestive Heart Failure (CHF)

In congestive heart failure, the heart fails to pump blood effectively. As a result, blood backs up. It can back up to the body (right-sided congestive heart failure) or the lungs (left-sided congestive heart failure).

1. *Causes:* Other illnesses can, over time, lead to congestive heart failure. These include hypertension; arrhythmias; diabetes; coronary artery disease; cardiomyopathy; emphysema; obesity; pulmonary embolism; anemia; and thyroid disease.
2. *Signs and symptoms*
   A. *Right-sided:* pitting pedal edema and jugular vein distention.
   B. *Left-sided:* crackles; shortness of breath; pulmonary edema (rales); tachypnea; distended jugular veins; and ventricular gallop.
3. *Interventions:* administer oxygen; establish IV access; monitor cardiac performance; and administer medications as ordered (e.g., furosemide, morphine, and nitroglycerin)

- Provide Foley catheter, bedside commode, or bedpan for frequent urination after furosemide.

Fast facts in a nutshell

Question: Which patient position is best to hear S3 (ventricular gallop), S4 (atrial gallop)?
Answer: *Left Lateral*

Notes: ______________________________

____

____

Acute Myocardial Infarction

Acute myocardial infarction is the result of a clogged coronary artery supplying blood to the heart muscle. The patient's history often reveals hypertension, coronary artery disease, high cholesterol, and smoking (see Figure 3.1).

1. *Causes:* blood clots; coronary arterial spasm from cocaine use. Contributing factors: hypertension; coronary artery disease; smoking; obesity; hyperlipidemia; and genetics.
2. *Signs and symptoms:* nausea and vomiting; diaphoresis; shortness of breath; and chest pain (described often as

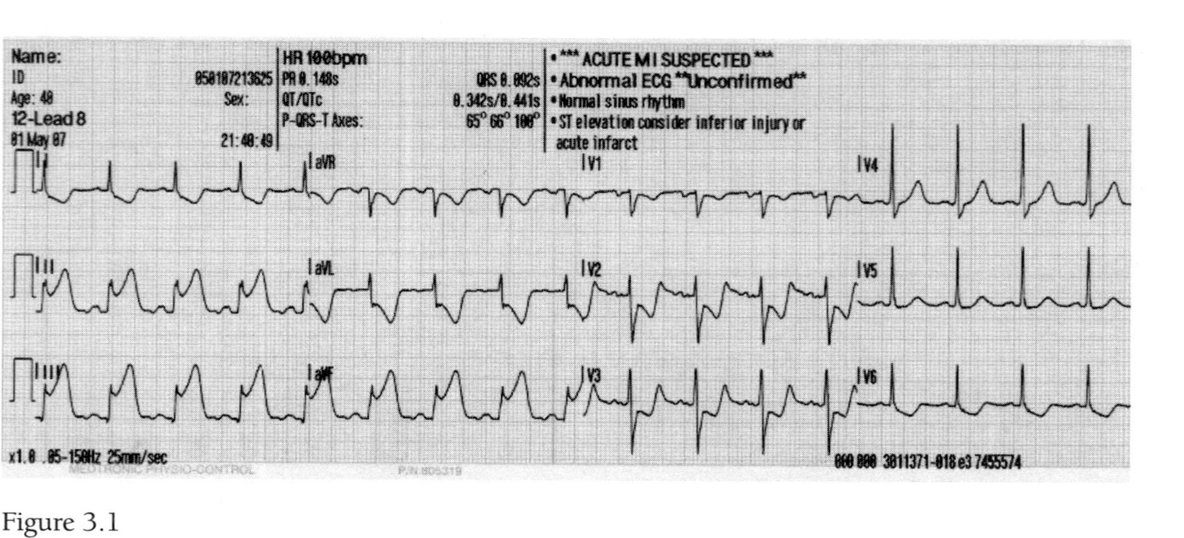
Name:
ID
Age: 48
12-Lead 8
01 May 07
050107213625
Sex:
21:40:49
HR 100bpm
PR 0.148s
QT/QTc
P-QRS-T Axes:
QRS 0.092s
0.342s/0.441s
65° 66° 100°
• *** ACUTE MI SUSPECTED ***
• Abnormal ECG **Unconfirmed**
• Normal sinus rhythm
• ST elevation consider inferior injury or acute infarct
I
aVR
V1
V4
III
aVL
V2
V5
III
aVF
V3
V6
x1.0 .05-150Hz 25mm/sec
000 000 3011371-018 e3 7455574

Figure 3.1

pressure, squeezing, tightness, or vague) that may radiate to the left shoulder or jaw.

3. *Interventions: MOVE*!!* (**M**onitor, **O**xygen, **V**enous access, and **E**KG); anticipate orders to: administer medications **MONA** (**m**orphine, **o**xygen, **n**itro SL, and **A**SA), obtain cardiac enzymes, arrange for chest X-ray, prepare for possible cardiac cath lab admission or thrombolytic or anticoagulant (heparin) therapy, and reassess/monitor chest pain.

Fast facts in a nutshell

Question: What factors absolutely contraindicate the use of thrombolytics?
Answer: *Active bleeding, recent surgery, or recent trauma.*

Question: What test should be done prior to administering heparin or thrombolytics?
Answer: *Hemoccult stool, coagulant studies.*

Question: What is the antidote for heparin?
Answer: *Protamine sulfate.*

Question: A patient allergic to shellfish might also be allergic to what medication?
Answer: *Protamine sulfate.*

Notes: ____________________

____

____

Arterial Occlusion

Arterial occlusion means a clogged artery.

1. *Causes:* coronary artery disease; atherosclerosis; hypertension; smoking; and hyperlipidemia.
2. *Signs and symptoms:* cool/pale extremities and weak pulse to the affected extremity.
3. *Interventions:* maintain extremity in dependent position; assess pulses through Doppler ultrasound; and prepare for possible surgery.

*Notes:*____

____

____

Endocarditis

Endocarditis is an infection to the inner lining of the heart and/or the heart valves.

1. *Causes:* Endocarditis occurs when a person with faulty heart valves contracts a common bacterial infection. For example, a bacterial infection in their skin can travel through the blood and attach to the faulty heart valve, resulting in endocarditis.
2. *Signs and symptoms:* chills; fever; splinter hemorrhaging of the nail beds; chest pain; and systolic murmur.

3. *Interventions:* administer antibiotics intravenously; obtain blood cultures and a complete blood count.

*Notes:*______________________________________

Aortic Injuries

Aortic injuries may occur anywhere on the ascending aorta, aortic arch, descending thoracic aorta, or abdominal aorta. The injuries can result in aneurysm, tear, or rupture. There is never enough time to repair a ruptured aorta. Without immediate surgery the patient can bleed to death rapidly. So it is critical for the nurse to identify an aortic injury early.

1. *Causes:* A history of aortic injuries may reveal hypertension; coronary artery disease; congestive heart failure; or a recent chest/abdominal trauma.
2. *Signs and symptoms* (may vary depending on location): hypotension; loss of consciousness; hypertension in upper extremities; stronger pulse in arms than legs; tearing chest pain that radiates to the back; tearing abdominal pain; chest wall ecchymosis; and paraplegia.
3. *Interventions:* get patient on a stretcher; obtain vital signs; check blood pressure in all extremities; notify provider of patient signs and symptoms immediately; prepare for immediate surgery; start two large-bore intravenous lines;

monitor cardiac performance; provide oxygen; perform electrocardiogram; and measure pulse oxygen.

Fast facts in a nutshell

Question: Which type of trauma most commonly causes a descending thoracic aortic laceration?
Answer: *Deceleration trauma that causes shearing.*

*Notes:*____

____

____

Symptomatic Bradycardia

Symptomatic bradycardia is a heart rate less than 60 beats per minute resulting in inadequate blood circulation. The patient is symptomatic, displaying signs of poor cardiac perfusion (see Figure 3.2).

1. *Causes:* The cause is not always known but underlying conditions such as coronary artery disease; heart disease; second or third degree heart blocks; hypertension; thyroid disease; and lung disease can contribute to bradycardia.
2. *Signs and symptoms:* heart rate lower than 60; patient looks and feels unwell (e.g., altered loss of consciousness, chest pain, diaphoretic, pale).

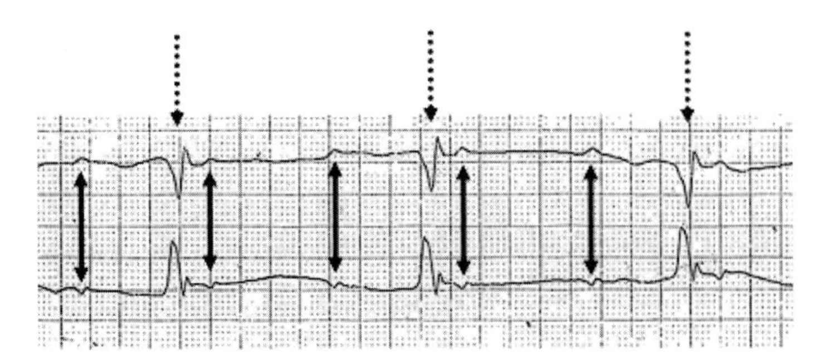

Figure 3.2

3. *Interventions:* assess ABCs; provide oxygen; check vital signs; measure pulse oxygen; perform electrocardiogram; monitor cardiac performance; anticipate orders to: intravenously push 0.5 to 1.0 mg of atropine at 3 to 5 minute intervals, establish transcutaneous pacing, administer medications (dopamine or epinephrine), and prepare for transvenous or interval pacer.

Notes: ____

____

____

Supraventricular Tachycardia (SVT)

In supraventricular tachycardia, the heart rate is regular but it beats at more than 150 beats per minute. Supraventricular tachycardia can be divided into symptomatic/unstable (patient

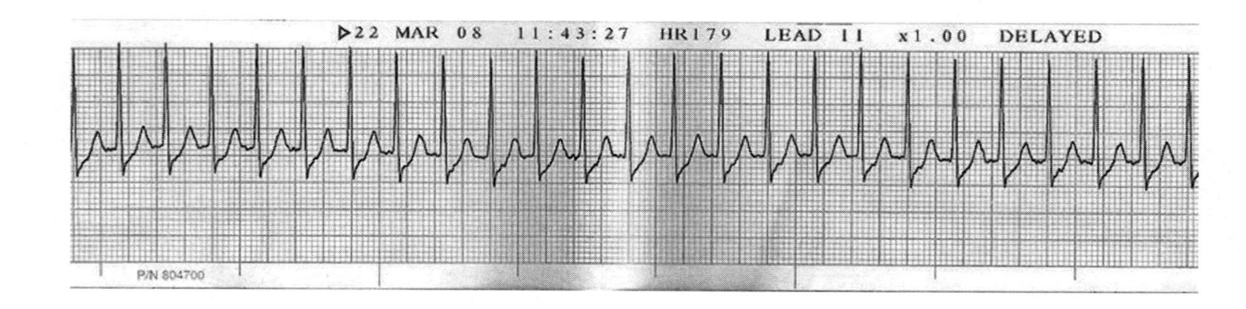

Figure 3.3

looks unwell) or asymptomatic/stable (patient looks fine). See Figure 3.3.

1. *Causes:* The cause is not always known. However, some habits and conditions can contribute to it, such as stress; caffeine; smoking; cocaine use; alcohol use; thyroid disease; heart failure; pulmonary embolism; chronic obstructive pulmonary disease; and pneumonia. Some medications for asthma, cold medications, and digoxin can also contribute to supraventricular tachcardia.
2. *Signs and symptoms:* palpitations; chest pain; diaphoresis; anxiety; and pulse rate greater than 150.
3. *Interventions:*
   A. *If patient is symptomatic and unstable:* anticipate order to: prepare for immediate synchronized cardioversion (100 j, 200 j, 300 j, 360 j, or biphasic equivalent).
   B. *If patient is asymptomatic and stable:* anticipate orders to: attempt vasovagal maneuvers, monitor cardiac performance, open large-bore intravenous line, provide oxygen, check vital signs, measure pulse oxygen, perform electrocardiogram, administer adenosine rapidly by intravenous push, and slow down atrial ventricle (AV) conduction with beta blockers/calcium channel blockers/digoxin or amiodarone.
      - Give patient a coffee straw and ask them to blow through it to assist vagal maneuvers.

Notes: ____

____

____

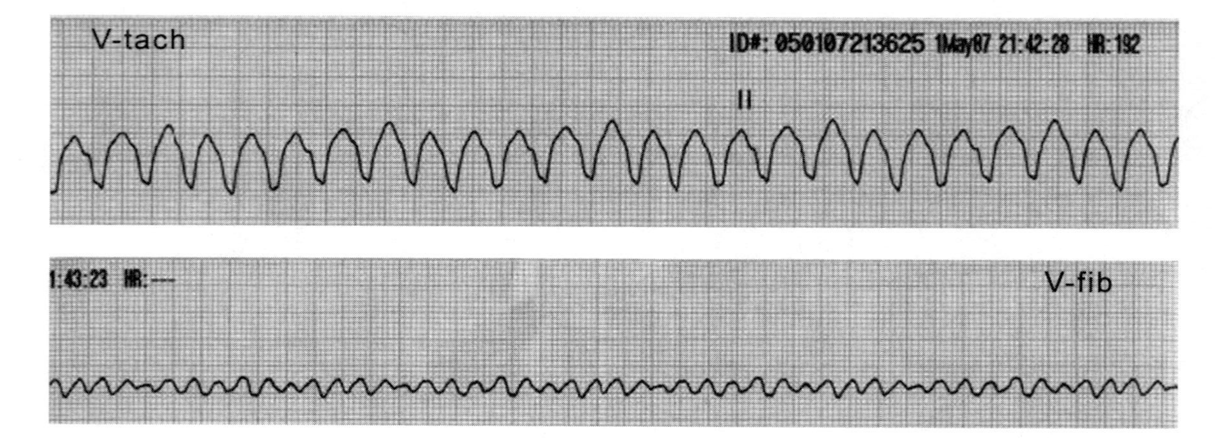

Figure 3.4

Ventricular Fibrillation or Pulseless Ventricular Tachycardia

Ventricular fibrillation and pulseless ventricular tachycardia are both irregular rapid rhythms in which there is no pulse. See Figure 3.4 and Table 3.1.

1. *Causes:* Poor cardiac perfusion due to coronary artery disease; shock; hypokalemia; myocardial infarct; or electrocution.
2. *Signs and symptoms:* decreased level of consciousness; no pulse; ventricular fibrillation or ventricular tachycardia on cardiac monitor.
3. *Interventions:* assess ABCs; open airway; assist breathing through bag valve mask or endotracheal tube; begin chest compressions while applying cardiac monitor/defibrillation

TABLE 3.1 Pulseless Ventricular Tachycardia or Ventricular Fibrillation Treatment

1) Shock at 120–200 j Biphasic or 360 j Monophasic
   - CPR 30/2 × 5 cycles or 2 min
   - Epinephrine 1 mg or Vasopressin 40 u IV/IO during CPR
2) Shock at 200 j Biphasic or 360 j Monophasic
   - CPR 30/2 × 5 cycles or 2 min
   - Amiodarone 300mg, 150mg 2nd dose or Lidocaine 1–1.5mg/kg, 0.5–0.75mg/kg 2nd dose during CPR
3) Shock at 200 j Biphasic or 360 j Monophasic
   - CPR 30/2 × 5 cycles or 2 min
   - Consider Magnesium 1–2 g IV/IO for Torsades de Pointes

pads; and DEFIBRILLATE! Just remember, shock then cardiopulmonary resuscitation (CPR) and **EV**eryone **S**tay **CALM**: **E**pinephrine or **V**asopressin, **S**hock, **CPR**, **A**miodarone or **L**idocaine, and **M**agnesium.

Fast facts in a nutshell

Question: If none of the above interventions work, what are some other causes of ventricular fibrillation?
Answer: *hypothermia, hypoxia, hypoglycemia, overdose, cardiac tamponade, tension pneumothorax, trauma, acidosis, hypovolemia, and electrolyte imbalances.*

Question: You see ventricular fibrillation on the monitor, but your patient is asymptomatic, sitting up, and talking to you. What is your first intervention?
Answer: *Check for a pulse. You can't believe everything you see on a monitor; it could be artifact.*

Question: What is the maximum number of times one can safely defibrillate a patient?
Answer: *There is no limit.*

Question: Why do we defibrillate?
Answer: *To temporarily produce asystole. This may sound incorrect, but debrillation actually depolarizes the heart, allowing the natural pacemakers of the heart to kick in.*

Question: Do precordal thumps work?
Answer: *Precordal thumps sometimes work and sometimes do not work. If you witness a true pulseless ventricular tachy-*

cardia/ventricular fibrillation, it only takes a second to administer precordal thumps while yelling for help. It might save a life.

Notes: ____

____

____

____

Pulseless Electrical Activity

Pulseless electrical activity occurs when a rhythm shows on the monitor, but the patient does not have a pulse. Again, you can't always believe what you see on the monitor.

1. *Causes:* can be attributed to the 5 Hs or 5 Ts.
   - Hypovolemia, Hypoxia, Hydrogen ion (acidosis), Hyper/hypokalemia, or Hypothermia
   - Toxin (drug overdose), Tamponade/cardiac, Tension Pneumothorax, Thrombosis, and Trauma
2. *Signs and symptoms:* Your patient has no pulse, but there is a rhythm on the monitor. Remember that just because there is electrical activity in the heart doesn't mean the heart is actually pumping.
3. *Interventions:* Check ABCs; perform cardiopulmonary resuscitation; per order, insert an intravenous line, monitor oxygen, administer medications (e.g., epinephrine and atropine).

Fast facts in a nutshell

Question: What is the effect of Nipride (nitroprusside) administered intravenously?
Answer: *It reduces afterload and increases cardiac output. It decreases myocardial oxygen demand without affecting the heart rate.*

Question: What type of electrocardiogram changes might you see in a patient with a potassium level of 7.8?
Answer: *bradycardia, peaked T waves, and widened QRS complex.*

Question: What equation defines cardiac output?
Answer: *heart rate × stroke volume*

Question: What are the manifestations of digoxin toxicity?
Answer: *blurred vision, halos, and arrhythmias.*

Question: What is the treatment for digoxin toxicity?
Answer: *glucagon, phenytoin (Dilantin), and digoxin immune fab (Digibind).*

Question: Name three vasopressors?
Answer: *Levophed, dopamine, and Aramine are vasopressors.*

Question: What dose of lidocaine should be administered to patients with renal failure, liver failure or patients who are elderly?
Answer: *Give half doses of lidocaine in patients with renal failure, liver failure, or who are elderly.*

Question: What is the antidote for warfarin (Coumadin)?
Answer: *Vitamin K.*

*Notes:*___

___

___

Fast facts in a nutshell

- Heparin affects partial thromboplastin time (PTT).
- Warfarin (Coumadin) affects prothrombin time (PT).

Fast facts in a nutshell: summary

Although cardiovascular diseases threaten lives every day, they can often be resolved with quick treatment. An emergency room nurse needs to understand the basics of cardiovascular assessments and treatments and be certified in advanced cardiovascular life support.

Chapter 4

Disaster Response Emergencies

INTRODUCTION

Working in the emergency department automatically makes you a first responder during a local disaster. Therefore, it is vital to know your role, communicate effectively, and locate equipment quickly. Disasters can be divided into two categories: natural and man-made. This chapter opens with the definitions, categories, and interventions for disasters. Many nurses may find remembering disaster instructions difficult because, quite simply, they are rarely used. Never fear. Just learn these three helpful mnemonics to remember what to do: **Disaster, MASS, and IDME.** *Then, the chapter guides you through some of the most common radiological, chemical, and biological exposures. Again, you may find it challenging to remember information that is used so infrequently, so just keep this book and the CDC Web site handy. Those two sources will provide all the information you need. To fully understand the material and ease your anxiety, be sure to practice an actual disaster drill in your facility during your orientation.*

During this part of your orientation, locate and become familiar with:

1. Your facility's disaster plans.
2. Your facility disaster codes.
3. Disaster/decontamination equipment.
4. Fire alarms and extinguishers.
5. Oxygen shut-off valves.
6. Evacuation plans and routes.
7. Contacts/whom to notify if a disaster occurs.
8. Where to sign up to participate in a disaster drill.
9. Disaster communication routes.
10. Personal Protective Equipment (PPE).

TYPES OF DISASTERS

A **disaster** is an event in which needs exceed resources. The types are indicated in Table 4.1.

INTERVENTIONS

To remember the proper interventions to follow in a disaster, remember the mnemonic, **DISASTER**, MASS, and IDME.

- Detect: What is the reason for the disaster. Are there mass casualties? Do our needs exceed our resources?
- Incident Command: People trained to manage, coordinate, and organize the disaster operation. Do we need them and, if so, where?

TABLE 4.1 Types of Disasters

Natural	Man-Made
Hurricane	Explosion
Earthquake	Fire
Landslide	Firearms
Ice storm/blizzard	Stampede
Fire	Structural collapse
Wildfire	Hazardous material
Flood	Power out
Tidal wave	Blocked communications
Tornado	Transportation event
Asteroid collision	• Airway (Plane)
Avalanche	• Railway (Train)
Volcanic eruption	• Waterway (Boat)
	• Roadway (Car)
	Weapons of mass destruction
	• Biological
	• Chemical
	• Nuclear

- Safe and Secure Scene: Is it safe? Always protect yourself and team members first, then the public, patients, and environment. Use personal protective equipment, such as gown, gloves, and masks.
- Assess Hazards: What are other potential hazards (for example, downed power lines, blood, smoke, leaking gas line, bad weather)?

- Support: What people and supplies are needed? Do we need HAZMAT team, fire and rescue team, law enforcement, vehicles, water?
- Triage and Treatment: Do we need triage? How much treatment is required? Follow your facilities disaster triage plan. If your facility does not have one, you can locate one online through FEMA.

MASS

- Move: Can the victims move? If so, they are less urgent. If they cannot, they are more urgent.
- Assess the victims who can't walk or move, as they are more urgent and need assistance.
- Sort victims using **IDME** or your current emergency department acuity scale.
  1. Immediate, Emergent, or Red acuity. They have an alteration in ABCs or threat to loss of life or limb.
  2. Delayed, Urgent, or Yellow acuity. These victims need medical attention, but they are not at risk of rapidly deteriorating.
  3. Minimal, Nonurgent, or Green. These victims have stable vital signs and minor wounds.
  4. Expectant or Blue. These victims have little or no chance of survival with current resources.

Send: immediate victims to hospitals/OR/ICU first.
Evacuate: Can the victims be transported to a safe location and, if so, how?
Recovery: What are some recovery issues?

Fast facts in a nutshell

To remember the proper interventions to follow in a disaster, remember the mnemonic, **DISASTER**, MASS, and IDME.

RADIATION, CHEMICAL, AND BIOLOGICAL EXPOSURES

Emergency medical personnel should always wear personal protective equipment, remove contaminated clothing, clean objects in 1% bleach solution, wash patient in proper decontamination showering systems, and report to infection control at the Centers for Disease Control at www.bt.cdc.gov (1-800-CDC-INFO).

Abrin or Ricin

Abrin or Ricin results from biological exposure to processed castor beans.

1. *Causes:* contact with poison released from processed castor beans, such as might occur at a castor bean plant. The poison inactivates type II ribosomes in the body.
2. *Signs and symptoms:* within a few days, metabolic acidosis; hepatitis; renal failure; and hematuria.

   a. *If poison is inhaled:* Within 4 to 8 hours, the patient will experience distress; fever; cough; shortness of breath; pulmonary edema; lung necrosis; and shock.
   b. *If poison is ingested:* nausea, vomiting, and diarrhea; rectal bleeding; hypotension; gastrointestinal necrosis; and hepatitis.
3. *Interventions:* decontaminate the patient with proper equipment; use standard precautions; administer fluids intravenously per order; and avoid exposure to contaminated substances. There is no antidote; treat the symptoms. Give charcoal, if ingestion is recent.

Notes: ______________________________

____

____

Anthrax

Anthrax is a spore-forming gram-positive bacteria (Bacillus anthracis). See Figure 4.1.

1. *Causes:* contaminated soil, animals, and animal products. The bacteria enter the body through inhalation, skin, or ingestion.
2. *Signs and symptoms*
   a. *If spore is inhaled:* Within 2 to 40+ days, flu-like symptoms, including weakness; cough; congestion; sore throat; fever; shortness of breath; respiratory distress; and shock

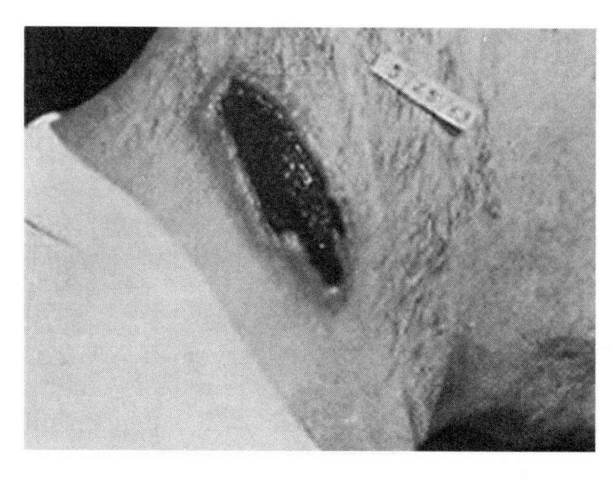

Figure 4.1

b. *If spore enters subcutaneously:* Within a week, an itchy vesicle turns into an ulcer and then a black scab, possibly with fever.
c. *If spore is ingested:* Within a week, nausea, vomiting, and diarrhea; rectal bleeding; and fever.

3. *Interventions:* anticipate orders to: obtain blood cultures, arrange for chest X-ray and CT scan, give antibiotics, like ciprofloxacin, and use standard precautions.

Fast facts in a nutshell

The inhaled form of anthrax has a very high fatality rate.

*Notes:*____

____

____

Botulism

Botulism is a paralyzing toxin produced by the bacteria Clostridium botulinum.

1. *Causes:* contaminated food; infected wounds; and spore consumption (e.g., honey) by infants.
2. *Signs and symptoms:* Within 4 days, patients have multiple cranial nerve palsies. The patient is also afebrile with bilateral facial droop; dysphonia; blurred vision; normal mental status; dry mouth; dysphagia; dysarthria; and bilateral descending skeletal muscle paralysis. Respiratory failure occurs in 24 hours or less.
3. *Interventions:* standard precautions; assess neurological status; monitor cardiac performance; measure pulse oxygen; collect gastric or stool samples; use ventilator if patient is experiencing respiratory failure; and give antitoxin available through state health departments and the Centers for Disease Control as ordered.

Fast facts in a nutshell

Question: An infant brought in to the emergency room for facial droop, muscle weakness, shallow respirations.

Botulism is suspected. What does this patient need from the Centers for Disease Control?
Answer: *Antitoxin.*

*Notes:*____

Blister Agent (Mustard Gas)

A blister agent is an alkaline agent with a mustard, onion, or garlic odor.

1. *Causes:* The gas is an agent used in chemical warfare that results in blisters and burns.
2. *Signs and symptoms:* Within 12 hours, the patient experiences second-degree burns; skin redness with blisters; corneal abrasions; sore throat; nausea, vomiting, and diarrhea; cough; and difficulty in breathing.
3. *Interventions:* decontaminate patient; perform ABCs first; treat symptoms, particularly chemical burns, with topical antibiotics as ordered. There is no antidote.

*Notes:*____

Brucellosis

Brucellosis is a bacterial (Brucella) infection.

1. *Causes:* infected animals or animal products.
2. *Signs and symptoms:* Within 4 weeks, the patient experiences fever; flu-like symptoms; sweating; headache; weakness; hepatitis; joint pain; arthritis; osteomyelitis; and endocarditis.
3. *Interventions:* use standard precautions; anticipate orders to: obtain blood cultures and give antibiotics (doxycycline, rifampin).

Notes: ____

____

____

Cyanide

Cyanide is a colorless chemical gas or crystal with a bitter almond odor.

1. *Causes:* Gas or crystals found in manufacturing, certain foods, and cigarette smoke.
2. *Signs and symptoms:* bradypnea; dizziness; weakness; headache; nausea; vomiting; tachycardia or bradycardia; hypotension; loss of consciousness; and respiratory failure.
3. *Interventions:* decontaminate patient; access and treat ABCs; and give cyanide antidote as ordered.

*Notes:*____

____

____

Nerve Agents

Nerve agents are chemical agents that block nerve impulses.

1. *Causes:* These agents can be absorbed through the skin or inhaled.
2. *Signs and symptoms:* remember SLUDGE (Saliva, Lacrimation, Urination, Defecation, GI upset, Emesis). Early symptoms include tachycardia; lethargy; paralysis; shock; anxiety; bronchospasms; ataxia; and pulmonary edema.
3. *Interventions:* decontaminate the patient. If the agent was ingested orally, anticipate order to: give 1 gm/kg of charcoal. Other orders may include: atropine to reverse central nervous system effects, Atrovent nebulizer to dry secretions, pralidoxime slowly over 30 minutes or obidoxime.

*Notes:*____

____

____

Plague (Bubonic)

Plague is a contagious bacterial infection (Yersinia pestis).

1. *Causes:* This bacterial infection is found endemically in animals. It spreads directly by infected flea bites to humans and other animals.
2. *Signs and symptoms:* Within 1 week, the patient experiences acute fever; chills; weakness; shortness of breath; hemoptysis; nausea, vomiting, and diarrhea; rapid and severe pneumonia; and sepsis.
3. *Interventions:* droplet precautions; anticipate orders to: obtain intravenous access, arrange for chest X-ray, collect blood and sputum cultures, and give antibiotics (streptomycin or gentamicin)

Fast facts in a nutshell

Question: How is the plague most commonly transmitted to humans?
Answer: *By* direct *contact with infected rodent fleas.*

*Notes:*______________________________________

Q-Fever

Q-fever is a Coxiella burnetii bacterial infection.

1. *Causes:* Coxiella burnetii bacteria found in animals and animal products.

2. *Signs and symptoms:* Within 2 to 3 weeks, the patient experiences flu-like symptoms (fever; cough; fatigue; nausea, vomiting, and diarrhea); abdominal pain; and hepatitis.
3. *Interventions:* maintain standard precautions, anticipate order to: give antibiotics (doxycycline, ciprofloxacin).

*Notes:*____

____

____

Radiation 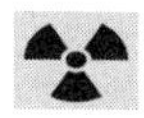

Radiation is a natural or manufactured form of energy that can be dangerous at high levels of exposure.

1. *Causes:* High-level exposures from sources such as a terrorist attack or nuclear power plant accident.
2. *Signs and symptoms:* burns; nausea; vomiting; diarrhea; weakness; bleeding; confusion; sepsis; or symptom free.
3. *Interventions:* provide medical personnel with radiation detection devices; use reverse isolation/neutropenic precautions; anticipate orders to: obtain a complete blood count, provide trauma/burn care, administer fluids intravenously, and give nausea medications and iodide tablets.

Fast facts in a nutshell

Question: An ER patient significantly exposed to radiation on the job will have which symptoms?
Answer: *Bloody diarrhea, nausea, and vomiting within 3 hours of radiation exposure.*

*Notes:*____

____

____

Smallpox

Smallpox is a viral infection (Variola major).

1. *Causes:* Spread by prolonged face-to-face contact; direct contact; or an exchange of bodily fluids.
2. *Signs and symptoms:* 2 to 3 days of fever; fatigue; nausea and vomiting; and delirium. This is followed by an approximately 4 to 6 mm macular rash on the face and extremities that turn to papules, vesicles, pustules, and finally scars.
3. *Interventions:* take airborne and contact precautions; place patient in negative pressure room; contact the Centers for Disease Control for laboratory testing and wound care; and give smallpox vaccination as ordered.

Fast facts in a nutshell

Smallpox has been successfully eradicated as a result of multinational vaccinations. Since people are no longer vaccinated, there is concern that the Variola major virus could be used as a bioterrorism weapon.

Notes: ____

____

____

Tularemia

Tularemia is a gram-negative bacterial infection (Franciscella tularensis).

1. *Causes:* spread by contact with infected animals, biting flies, or ticks.
2. *Signs and symptoms:* Within 2 weeks, the patient experiences abdominal pain; fever; nausea, vomiting, and diarrhea; pneumonia; conjunctivitis; skin ulcer; and lymphadenitis.
3. *Interventions:* establish droplet precautions; gather blood or sputum cultures; and give antibiotics (ciprofloxacin, doxycycline, gentamicin) as ordered.

*Notes:*____

Viral Hemorrhagic Fevers

Viral hemorrhagic fevers include infections, such as Ebola, Marburg, and yellow fever.

1. *Causes:* spread by inhalation, direct contact, or bodily fluid exchange.
2. *Signs and symptoms:* Within 3 weeks, the patient experiences fever; petechial rash; jaundice; disseminated intravascular coagulation; hepatitis; and renal failure.
3. *Interventions:* establish airborne/contact precautions; anticipate orders to: obtain a complete blood count, perform liver function tests, check prothrombin/partial thromboplastin time, place patient in negative pressure room, and give antivirals, such as arenavirus or ribavirin. Medical personnel require full body personal protective equipment and personal air purifying respirators. Yellow fever vaccine is available, but the infection takes over before the vaccine is effective.

*Notes:*____

Cholera (Vibrio cholerae)

Cholera, an intestinal infection caused by the bacterium Vibrio cholerae, is uncommon in the United States, but may occur in individuals who return home after travel to Africa, India, or South America. Its severe state can be life-threatening from rapid loss of body fluids and shock.

1. *Causes:* spreads through ingested fecal-contaminated water or food.
2. *Signs and symptoms:* severe watery diarrhea and vomiting; leg cramps; dehydration; and shock.
3. *Interventions:* maintain standard precautions; anticipate orders to: perform a complete blood count and basic metabolic panel, provide fluid bolus intravenously, and possibly give antibiotics.

*Notes:*____

____

____

Fast facts in a nutshell: summary

Disasters are rarely predictable and are always chaotic. So, it is critical that you be prepared and know the plan of action for your facility. Become familiar with all available disaster equipment. Although this chapter should give you a good working knowledge of common forms of disasters and what to do, participating in disaster drills is an essential piece of the puzzle. Be sure to routinely refresh your disaster nursing skills.

Chapter 5

Ear, Nose, and Throat (ENT) Emergencies

INTRODUCTION

Ear, nose, and throat emergencies are daily occurrences in the emergency room. ***Most of the time, they are not life-threatening.*** *From foreign objects to trauma or infection, this chapter will take you through the most common ear, nose, and throat emergencies you will face. For each emergency, you will learn causes, manifestations, and interventions.*

During this part of your orientation, you should locate and become familiar with:

1. Alligator forceps.
2. Ear wicks.
3. Eardrops for infection and cerumen impaction.
4. Ear irrigation supplies, ear curettes.

5. Head lamp.
6. Nasal packing supplies.

DIAGNOSES

Foreign Objects

You name it; it can be found in an ear or a nostril. Commonly occurs with curious young children and toddlers, but occasionally with adult patients. Hopefully, the object will be detected before infection occurs. Getting it out of the uncooperative 3-year-old patient is the real trick!

1. *Causes:* Foreign object in the ear, such as nuts, bolts, raisins, peas, beads, bugs, and cotton.
2. *Signs and symptoms:* visible foreign object; purulent or bloody discharge; discomfort or pain; swelling; redness; foul odor; and foreign body sensation.
3. *Interventions*
   A. Remove the foreign body with suction, irrigation, alligator forceps, or ear curette. Provide ear antibiotics or nasal decongestants as ordered. Instruct the patient not to put anything smaller than an elbow in his or her ears or nose!
   B. Sometimes nasal foreign bodies can be dislodged simply by closing off the unaffected nostril and asking the patient to blow forcefully out of the affected nostril.
   C. If unable to remove foreign body, provider may refer patient to ear, nose, and throat specialist.

Fast facts in a nutshell

There are many ways to flush an ear, but this seems to work the best for wax removal.

1. First, gather lukewarm water with a splash of peroxide mixed in a small basin and a 20-ml syringe with plastic needle-less short tip. You can also cut off the end of an intravenous catheter.
2. Lay the patient on his/her side with affected ear up. Fill the ear canal with warm water and peroxide solution and let soak for 10 minutes. Then sit patient up with basin under ear to catch fluids. Now that the wax is softened, irrigate ear canal using syringe and rest of water solution. If a brown scaly pebble comes out, this is the wax impaction; you got it!

Notes: ______________________________

____

____

Acute Otitis Externa (Swimmer's Ear)

Acute otitis externa is a bacterial or fungal infection of the outer ear.

1. *Causes:* Outer ear infections commonly occur because of frequent swimming or foreign objects in the ear. Bacteria or fungus enter with the water or the foreign object, thereby causing an infection.
2. *Signs and symptoms:* outer ear pain; itchy, impaired hearing; ear discharge; fever; erythema; and swelling of the outer ear.
3. *Interventions:* give topical eardrop solution/antibiotics as ordered; provide ear wick; and use warm compresses. Instruct the patient not to swim until the infection is resolved (7–10 days).

Fast facts in a nutshell

- When examining the ear in an adult, pull *up* and back, in a child under three years of age, pull the ear *down* and back.
- Avulsed teeth should be placed in cold milk, ice water, or replaced in conscious patient's mouth within 30 minutes.

Notes: ______________________________

____

____

____

Acute Otitis Media

Acute otitis media is a middle ear bacterial or viral infection. It is more common in children because of their short, narrow eustachian tubes. An infant or toddler with otitis media may appear irritable, be crying, pulling at ears, and have a poor appetite, nausea, vomiting, or diarrhea.

1. *Causes:* Middle ear infections usually start as a sinus infection.
2. *Signs & symptoms:* recent upper respiratory infection; earache; impaired hearing; red or dull gray bulging tympanic membrane; and fever.
3. *Interventions:* administer and evaluate effectiveness of antipyretics, antibiotics, and pain medication such as Auralgan, as ordered.

*Notes:*____________________________________

____

____

Ruptured Tympanic Membrane

This is a tear or rupture of the tympanic membrane (eardrum).

1. *Causes:* Tears may be the result of infection or trauma from a foreign object (Q-tip, bobby pin) or other forces (e.g., explosions, skull fractures, burns).
2. *Signs and symptoms:* ear pain; discharge; impaired hearing; vertigo; nausea, vomiting, and fever.

3. *Interventions:* With most small perforations, the eardrum grows back on its own, similar to the way a fingernail grows back. Anticipate orders to: administer oral antibiotics, prepare for surgery in large perforations, instruct patient not to blow nose or get ears wet, and provide follow-up with an ear, nose, and throat specialist.

Notes: ____

____

____

Ménière's disease

Ménière's disease is an inner ear disorder affecting adults between 40 and 50 years of age.

1. *Causes:* Its cause is unknown. Symptoms usually occur suddenly and can last from a few minutes to a few hours.
2. *Signs and symptoms:* vertigo; dizziness; nausea and vomiting; tinnitus; impaired hearing; diaphoresis; headache; and blurred vision.
3. *Interventions:* bring side rails up (fall precautions) and put the bed in the low locked position; speak slow and clearly; administer Valium (intravenously) for rapid relief and antiemetics as ordered; require bedrest and a quiet environment; and provide diet instructions (low sodium, no caffeine, and no nicotine).

*Notes:*____

____

____

Allergic Rhinitis (Hay Fever)

Rhinitis is a nasal mucous membrane inflammation.

1. *Causes:* allergic response to pollen, dust, or other allergens. It may be acute (seasonal) or chronic (perennial).
2. *Signs and symptoms:* watery nasal drainage; nasal congestion; sneezing; cough; and sore throat. Infants may present with difficulty breathing or poor feeding.
3. *Interventions:* administer medications as ordered (analgesics, antibiotics, decongestants, antihistamines); increase fluid intake; and perform bulb syringe suction in infants.

*Notes:*____

____

____

Epistaxis

Epistaxis is a nose bleed. There are two types: anterior bleeds and posterior bleeds.

Anterior bleeds are more common and easier to control.

1. *Causes:* trauma; cocaine use; disease; nose picking; or just dry air during winter months.
2. *Signs and symptoms:* bright red nasal bleeding.
3. *Interventions:* position patient sitting up and leaning forward; apply direct pressure to bridge of nose; apply ice; administer medications as ordered (pseudoephedrine); and prepare for cauterization or nasal packing.

Posterior bleeds are less common and more difficult to control.

1. *Causes:* Usually associated with chronic medical problems, such as hypertension, blood dyscrasia, or tumor.
2. *Signs and symptoms:* nasal bleeding.
3. *Interventions:* apply direct pressure and ice for 10 minutes or more. Position the patient sitting up leaning forward over a large basin. Establish large-bore intravenous access if ordered; have suction and head lamp available; arrange for ear, nose, and throat consult as ordered; prepare for procedure (posterior nasal packing, nasal tampon, or cauterization); and monitor level of consciousness, vital signs, pulse oxygen, and bleeding. *Instruct patient not to blow nose.*

Notes: ____

____

____

Nasal Fracture

This is a fracture of the nasal bones.

1. *Causes:* direct trauma to the nose.
2. *Signs and symptoms:* nasal bleeding; nasal ecchymosis or edema; nasal airway obstruction; and deformity or tenderness over nasal bridge.
3. *Interventions:* control bleeding with direct pressure; apply ice; administer analgesics as ordered and evaluate effectiveness; and arrange for nasal or facial X-ray. *Instruct patient not to blow nose.*
   - If nasal airway is not obstructed, no treatment is necessary.
   - If nasal airway is obstructed, patient will be referred to an ear, nose, and throat specialist for repair *one week after swelling decreases.*

*Notes:*____

____

____

Sinusitis

Sinusitis is a sinus inflammation.

1. *Causes:* infection; allergies; chemical irritants; pressure changes; cocaine use; dental abscesses; or mechanical obstruction.
2. *Signs and symptoms:* pain; purulent nasal drainage; and fever.
3. *Interventions:* anticipate order to: administer medications and evaluate effectiveness (decongestants, antibiotic, analgesic/narcotic) and arrange for sinus films or CT scan.

*Notes:*____

Pharyngitis/Tonsillitis

This is inflammation of the throat or tonsils.

1. *Causes:* bacterial or viral infection.
2. *Signs and symptoms:* sore throat; red swollen tonsils; white pus on tonsils; difficulty swallowing; fever; ear pain; foul breath; and swollen cervical lymph nodes.
3. *Interventions:* arrange for strep or monospot test; administer antibiotic by mouth (PO) or injection (IM) as ordered; and monitor airway patency.
   - Soft tissue neck X-ray may be used to rule out *epiglottitis* or retropharyngeal abscess when patient demonstrates pain; drooling; "hot-potato voice"; or difficulty breathing.

*Notes:*____

Peritonsillar Abscess

This is an abscess of the tonsil. It may be a respiratory emergency if the airway is obstructed.

1. *Causes:* commonly caused by streptococcus bacteria
2. *Signs and symptoms:* sore throat; unilateral swollen tonsil; swollen cervical lymph nodes; dysphagia; fever; difficulty opening mouth; swollen palate; laterally displaced uvula; drooling; and muffled or "hot-potato voice."
3. *Interventions:* prepare for incision and drainage of abscess with ear, nose, and throat consultant; administer antibiotics and pulse oxygen; and monitor airway.

Fast facts in a nutshell

Question: What is the difference between tonsillitis and peritonsillar abscess?
Answer: *With tonsillitis, both tonsils are swollen. With peritonsillar abscess, one tonsil is swollen.*

*Notes:*____

____

____

Fast facts in a nutshell: summary

You should now have a basic understanding of the ear, nose, and throat problems that are seen daily in the emergency room. Don't be afraid to take an otoscope and assess your patient's ears, nose, or throat. Most providers appreciate a good assessment, especially one that is well documented before and after treatment.

Chapter 6

Fluid and Electrolyte Imbalances

INTRODUCTION

*As you already may know, **a fluid and electrolyte balance is essential to maintaining homeostasis within the body.** If not treated, interruptions to this balance can be fatal. Therefore, it is vital for the emergency room nurse to recognize the the most common manifestations of fluid and electrolyte imbalances and how to correct them quickly.*

During this part of your orientation, locate and become familiar with:

1. Doppler machine for pedal pulses.
2. Peritoneal centesis tray and fluid containers.
3. Medications: furosemide, potassium intravenously and by mouth, calcium chloride, calcium gluconate, sodium bicarbonate, magnesium sulfate, dextrose with intravenous regular insulin, Kayexalate, glucocorticoids, phosphate, calcitonin, and ethylenediamine tetra acetic acid.

4. Intravenous fluids: normal saline (0.9%), or 0.3% if severe, Ringer's Lactate (RL), D_5W (dextrose 5% in water), and D_5NS (dextrose 5% in 0.45% normal saline).
5. Lab values: sodium, potassium, calcium, phosphorus, magnesium.

DIAGNOSES

Edema

Edema occurs when plasma fluid shifts into the interstitial space. There are four different types of edema based on location and injury.

Pulmonary edema: fluid shifts to the lungs.

1. *Causes:* left-sided congestive heart failure; chest trauma; anaphylactic shock; and septic shock.
2. *Signs and symptoms:* shortness of breath, jugular vein distention (JVD), and crackle breath sounds.
3. *Interventions:* anticipate orders to: arrange for chest X-ray, provide oxygen, and give diuretics (furosemide).

Ascites: fluid shifts to the abdomen.

1. *Causes:* liver problems or abdominal trauma.
2. *Signs and symptoms:* abdominal swelling/edema. The patient may also have pedal edema.
3. *Interventions:* anticipate patient will receive a peritoneocentesis and other measures to correct underlying liver problems.

Pedal edema: fluid shifts to the lower extremities.

1. *Causes:* right-sided congestive heart failure; lower extremity trauma; peripheral vascular disease; cast applied too tightly; high sodium diet; and lymphedema.
2. *Signs and symptoms:* feet swelling and edema.
3. *Interventions:* give diuretic as ordered (furosemide); assess pedal pulses; and document stage of edema.

Severe burns: fluid shifts to burned areas causing localized edema.

1. *Causes:* The body's natural response to a severe burn injury is swelling and fluid shift.
2. *Signs and symptoms:* localized edema to area of burn.
3. *Interventions:* volume replacement. Patient is experiencing cellular dehydration.

*Notes:*____

____

____

Hyponatremia

Hyponatremia is a sodium level below 135.

1. *Causes:* Syndrome of inappropriate antidiuretic hormone, medications (morphine sulfate, penicillin G, barbiturates, diuretics, and oxytocin), too much D_5W; nausea, vomiting, and diarrhea; gastrointestinal suction; excessive sweating; Addison's disease; extracellular fluid

loss (burns, peritonitis, bowel obstruction); and congestive heart failure.

2. *Signs and symptoms:* irritability; nausea and vomiting; seizures; weakness; orthostatic hypotension; headache; tachycardia; lethargy; abdominal cramps; and dry oral mucosa.
3. *Interventions:* anticipate orders to: correct fluid imbalances, intravenously administer normal saline 0.9% or 0.3% if hyponatremia is severe, perform basic metabolic panel, and monitor closely.

Notes: ____________________________________

____

____

Hypernatremia

Hypernatremia is a sodium level above 145.

1. *Causes:* diabetes insipidus; poor fluid intake in hot weather; fever; infections; renal disease; diarrhea; excessive sweating; diaphoresis; overly effective diuretics; and burns.
2. *Signs and symptoms:* anorexia; nausea; vomiting; agitation; thirst; oliguria; seizure; lethargy; coma; and muscle weakness/twitching.
3. *Interventions:* anticipate order to give water by mouth or to start an intravenous line for intravenous rehydration.

Notes: ____________________________________

____

____

Hypokalemia

Hypokalemia is a potassium level below 3.5.

1. *Causes:* burns; gastrointestinal obstruction; acute alcoholism; diuretics; Cushing's syndrome (adrenal hyperactivity); nausea, vomiting, and diarrhea; uncontrolled diabetes mellitus; excessive sweating; or gastrointestinal suctioning.
2. *Signs and symptoms:* lethargy; fatigue; muscle weakness and decreased/absent deep tendon reflexes; tachycardia; paralysis; paralytic ileus; weak irregular pulse; tetany; orthostatic hypotension; and flatten/inverted T wave on an electrocardiogram.
3. *Interventions:* anticipate orders to: correct alkalosis (no sodium bicarbonate, no vomiting, no diarrhea, and no gastrointestinal suctioning), administer potassium by mouth or intravenously, perform basic metabolic panel, check magnesium, and give intravenous lactated Ringer's fluids.

Fast facts in a nutshell

- The correct rate of infusion of an intravenous potassium drip is no faster than 20 mEq of potassium chloride per hour on a pump.
- If infused too quickly, it can cause fatal arrhythmias and phlebitis!

*Notes:*________________________________

Hyperkalemia

Hyperkalemia is a potassium level above 4.5.

1. *Causes:* renal failure; diabetes mellitus; tissue trauma; early burn stages; excessive potassium intake; potassium-sparing diuretics; hyponatremia; and respiratory/metabolic acidosis.
2. *Signs and symptoms:* muscle weakness, cramps, and pain; peaked T-waves and depressed ST segments on electrocardiogram; nausea, vomiting, and diarrhea; paresthesia; irritability; and dysrhythmias; sinus bradycardia; first-degree heart block; ventricular fibrillation; and asystole.
3. *Interventions:* anticipate orders to: monitor cardiac performance, restrict potassium intake (in food or medication), administer normal saline bolus intravenously, and give diuretics, Kayexalate by mouth or rectum, calcium chloride or calcium gluconate, sodium bicarbonate, and intravenous regular insulin with intravenous glucose (D_{50}).

Figure 6.1 illustrates electrocardiogram changes during hypokalemia and hyperkalemia. You can see how potassium directly affects the heart.

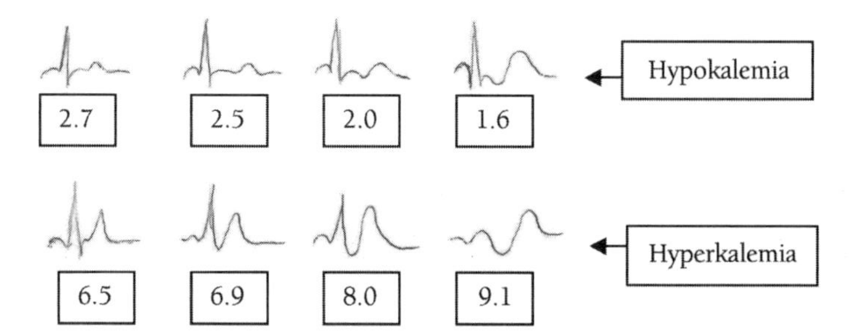

Figure 6.1

Fast facts in a nutshell

- It is normal to have a high potassium level with a high blood sugar.
- As the blood sugar decreases with insulin treatment, the potassium will shift into the cell, and the serum potassium level will drop.

*Notes:*____

Hypocalcemia

Hypocalcemia is a calcium level below 8.5. It leads to increased neuromuscular excitability.

1. *Causes:* lack of parathyroid hormone; vitamin D deficiency; peritonitis; bone cancer; calcium channel blocker overdose; pancreatitis; burns; sepsis; shock; trauma; alcoholism; and malnutrition.
2. *Signs and symptoms:* anxiety; irritability; seizure; nausea, vomiting, and diarrhea; muscle cramps; tetany; dysrhythmias; unconsciousness; and cardiac failure.
   - Chvostek's sign: facial muscle spasms when facial nerve tapped anterior to external ear below the temporal bone.
   - Trousseau's sign: Hand/carpal spasms when pumping up BP cuff above systolic pressure for three minutes.
3. *Interventions:* anticipate orders to: administer normal saline intravenously, monitor cardiac performance, give calcium chloride or calcium gluconate intravenously, and correct magnesium deficit.

*Notes:*____

____

____

Hypercalcemia

Hypercalcemia is a calcium level above 10.6. It leads to decreased neuromuscular excitability.

1. *Causes:* renal disease; hyperparathyroidism; too much vitamin D; drinking too much milk; pancreatitis; peptic ulcers; thiazide diuretics; and prolonged immobilization.
2. *Signs and symptoms:* muscle weakness; dehydration; nausea and vomiting; constipation; ileus; kidney stones; lethargy;

headache; irritability; decreased level of consciousness; dysrhythmias (short QT interval); and cardiac arrest.

3. *Interventions:* anticipate orders to: administer diuretics and 1 to 2 liters of normal saline bolus intravenously, monitor cardiac rhythm, perform basic metabolic panel, measure magnesium level, measure intake and output, monitor for cardiac heart failure, and administer medications (glucocorticoids, calcitonin, phosphate, or ethylenediamine tetra acetic acid).

*Notes:*____

____

____

Overhydration

Overhydration is also known as fluid overload.

1. *Causes:* drinking too much water or fluids. Receiving too much intravenous fluid.
2. *Signs and symptoms:* pedal/pulmonary edema; nausea and vomiting; headache; anorexia; confusion; seizure; aphasia; or blurred vision.
3. *Interventions:* anticipate orders to: restrict fluids, give diuretics, monitor intake and output, and check level of consciousness.

*Notes:*____

____

____

Dehydration

Dehydration is a lack of fluids.

1. *Causes:* inadequate fluid intake; fever; excessive sweating; and vomiting or diarrhea.
2. *Signs and symptoms:* confusion; disorientation; seizure; dry oral mucosa; dry skin; hyperthermia; weak rapid pulse; orthostatic hypotension; orthostasis; lethargy; fever; thirst; sunken fontanelles and eyes in infants; lack of tears in crying children; concentrated urine; tachypnea; tachycardia; and decreased urine output.
3. *Interventions:* anticipate orders to: give fluids intravenously or by mouth, administer antipyretics for fever, perform basic metabolic panel and electrocardiogram, assess mental status, check orthostatic vital signs, and measure intake and output.

*Notes:*____________________________________

____

____

Hyperosmolar Hyperglycemic Nonketotic Coma (HHNC)

This is a severe state of dehydration as a result of a very high blood sugar count (greater than 600, but usually in the 1000s).

1. *Causes:* The high level of sugar results in very thick blood, so the body tries to void the sugar. The process of frequent voiding, however, results in excessive loss of body fluids.

2. *Signs and symptoms:* Imagine a shriveled dried-up raisin, as this is your HHNC patient. Look for thirst; warm and dry skin; hemiparesis; urinary frequency; weakness; change in level of consciousness; seizure; tachycardia; fever; and absence of ketones in urine.
3. *Interventions:* These patients need about 9 liters of intravenous fluids. Anticipate orders to: start with normal saline intravenous bolus, and then change the intravenous fluid to 5% Dextrose 0.45% normal saline (D5 ½ NS) once the blood sugar is less than 300; administer regular insulin at 5 to 10 units intravenous push, followed by a drip of 0.05 units/kg/hr until blood sugar is less than 300, monitor cardiac rhythm, perform electrocardiogram, check blood sugar every hour, prepare a complete blood count, basic metabolic panel, and urinalysis, replace potassium, and prepare for intensive care unit admission.

Fast facts in a nutshell

Note the symptom and blood sugar differences between hyperosmolar hyperglycemic nonketotic coma and diabetic ketoacidosis.

- Hyperglycemic nonketotic coma means that blood sugar is very high (600 to 1000s). Patient is severely dehydrated, and there are *no* ketones in the urine.
- Diabetic ketoacidosis blood sugar is moderately high (300 to 600). The patient may be mildly dehydrated, and ketones are present in the urine.

*Notes:*____

____

____

Fast facts in a nutshell: summary

Fluids and electrolytes play a key role in health and homeostasis. It is critical that emergency room nurses understand this delicate balance, as a slight disturbance in this amazing balance can be fatal. Make sure you learn the different lab values, for you will need them every day in evaluating a wide variety of illnesses.

Chapter 7

Gastrointestinal Emergencies

INTRODUCTION

The gastrointestinal system is made up of several organs, including the stomach, liver, pancreas, gallbladder, and intestines. Gastrointestinal emergencies can be a very messy everyday emergency room occurrence. Ruptured bowels, vomiting, diarrhea, constipation, enemas, you name it; you will see all types of gastrointestinal problems in the emergency room. Catching the projectile vomit in the basin is the real trick! After reviewing this chapter, you will be able to differentiate the types of gastrointestinal emergencies, their causes, manifestations, and treatments. ***For each patient, prepare a full gastrointestinal assessment and document it thoroughly.***

During this part of your orientation, locate and become familiar with:

1. Suction equipment.
2. Gastric lavage equipment and nasogastric tubes.
3. Hemoccult and gastrocult specimens.

4. Enemas.
5. Basins, Chux, and incontinence pads or liners.
6. Medications to know: gastrointestinal (GI) cocktail, famotidine (Pepcid), pantoprazole (Protonix), promethazine (Phenergan), metoclopramide (Reglan), and ondansetron hydrochloride (Zofran).

NEVER UNDERESTIMATE ABDOMINAL PAIN

I once had a female patient come in by ambulance complaining of abdominal pain for 5 minutes. I thought it was a little silly to call an ambulance after just 5 minutes of pain. She was hollering, wailing, and carrying on so much that I could barely get a history. She was seen, assessed by a doctor, and X-rayed in about 15 minutes. Then she said her chest hurt. It turned out she not only had a ruptured bowel, but she also was having an acute myocardial infarction at the same time! Boy, were we shocked! So, although a patient may appear to be just very dramatic, **never underestimate abdominal pain.**

Fast facts in a nutshell

- A patient who has vomited 20 times in the last 8 hours is at risk for **metabolic alkalosis and hypokalemia.**
- After ingesting bleach, the patient has corrosive injury to the esophagus. Initial assessment and treatment should include **airway management.**
- Causes of ascites include **constrictive pericarditis, cirrhosis, and peritonitis.**

- The abdomen is assessed in which order? **Inspection, Auscultation, Percussion, and Palpation (look, listen, and feel).**
- **Sepsis** is the most common problem associated with colon trauma.

*Notes:*____

____

____

DIAGNOSES

Gastritis

Gastritis is an inflammation of the stomach lining that can be an acute or chronic condition. Chronic gastritis can lead to ulcers and gastrointestinal bleeding.

1. *Causes:* infection; stress; gastroesophageal reflux disease; aspirin; alcohol; or food poisoning.
2. *Signs and symptoms:* nausea and vomiting; gastrointestinal bleeding; pain; malaise; anorexia; and loss of appetite.
3. *Interventions:* anticipate orders to: administer fluids intravenously, arrange for abdominal X-ray, provide blood if severe blood loss, prepare a complete blood count and basic metabolic panel, and administer medications (e.g., antacids, gastrointestinal cocktail, histamine receptor antagonists, and antiemetics).

Fast facts in a nutshell

A gastrointestinal cocktail is made up of *Maalox and belladonna (adding 10 milliliters of viscous lidocaine makes it a super gastrointestinal cocktail).*

Fast facts in a nutshell

Question: A 36-year-old male patient complains of burning epigastric pain 1 to 2 hours after eating for 1 to 2 weeks. What is your diagnosis?
Answer: *peptic ulcer disease.*

Gastroenteritis

Gastroenteritis is an inflammation of the stomach or small intestine. It is often the diagnosis when the patient says, "I think I have the stomach flu."

1. *Causes:* viruses; bacteria; parasites; toxins; or allergens. The most common viruses that cause gastroenteritis are *Norwalk virus and Rotavirus.*
2. *Signs and symptoms:* nausea, vomiting, and diarrhea; abdominal pain or cramps; fever; dehydration; and hypovolemia in the very young or very old.

3. *Interventions:* anticipate orders to: provide fluids intravenously, prepare a basic metabolic panel and complete blood count, administer medications (antibiotics, antiparasitic agents), and provide patient education on a clear liquid and BRAT (bananas, rice, applesauce, and toast) diet.
   - Discharge teaching should include avoiding meat and dairy products, spicy foods, alcohol, greasy foods, and acidic foods.
   - Infants should not stop formula feeding for more than 24 hours.
   - Recovering from nausea and vomiting is a gradual process. The patient should have nothing by mouth for an hour or so after vomiting. Then clear liquids should be introduced in small increments (ice chips) for 24 hours, after which the patient can advance to full liquids. The next step is BRAT diet. Finally, the advanced diet as tolerated. Follow this process gradually or you'll be cleaning up vomit!

*Notes:*____

____

____

Gastroesophageal Reflux Disease (GERD)

Gastroesophageal reflux disease is commonly called acid reflux. It occurs when excess stomach acid travels up the esophagus, resulting in esophagitis.

1. *Causes:* The malfunction of the esophageal sphincter and hiatal hernia are the major causes. Contributing factors are cigarette smoking; lying down after meals; and consuming alcohol, large meals, spicy or acidic food, and caffeine.
2. *Signs and symptoms:* upper midsternal burning pain and indigestion.
3. *Interventions:* anticipate orders for: antacids and gastrointestinal cocktail. Educate the patient to avoid fatty or fried foods, chocolate, alcohol, and overeating. The patient should not lie down for three hours after eating.

*Notes:*____

____

____

Intestinal Obstruction

This is the inability to move gastrointestinal contents through intestines. The two types of obstructions: large bowel and small bowel. As the nurse, you will prefer to treat the patient with the large bowel obstruction, because nothing is coming out of either end. On the other hand, the patient with small bowel obstruction will be vomiting and having diarrhea. You will need plenty of bedpans and emesis basins.

1. *Causes:* adhesions; hernia; volvulus; intussusception; tumor; paralytic ileus; mesenteric infarction; and abdominal angina.

2. *Signs and symptoms:* fever; abdominal distention; nausea and vomiting; rapid onset of abdominal pain; dehydration; weight loss or weight gain (due to fluid retention); high-pitched or absent bowel sounds; and constipation or recent diarrhea.
3. *Interventions:* anticipate orders to: arrange for abdominal CT scan or X-rays, monitor orthostatic vital signs, give nothing by mouth, administer fluids intravenously, use nasogastric tube for gastric decompression, and administer antibiotic medications.

Fast facts in a nutshell

Tips for nasogastric tube insertion:

1. Be nice when inserting a tube down a patient's *belly;* use lidocaine *jelly* to lubricate the tip.
2. Oral anesthetic spray to the throat.
3. Check placement initially by *auscultating stomach, confirming that the patient is able to speak, and checking gastric content.*
4. To help the tube curve down the nasopharynx, curl the tip of the nasogastric tube around your finger first.

Notes: ______________________________

____

____

Appendicitis

Appendicitis is an inflammation of the appendix. If it ruptures, it could lead to peritonitis, sepsis, and then septic shock!

1. *Causes:* stomach virus or food particles trapped in the appendix.
2. *Signs and symptoms:* constant dull right lower quadrant; abdominal pain (McBurney's Point; see Figure 7.1); rebound tenderness; nausea, vomiting and diarrhea/constipation; low-grade fever (usually after first 24 hours); and manifestations of peritonitis (fever, guarding, abdominal pain and distention, hypoactive bowel sounds, and diffuse rigidity).

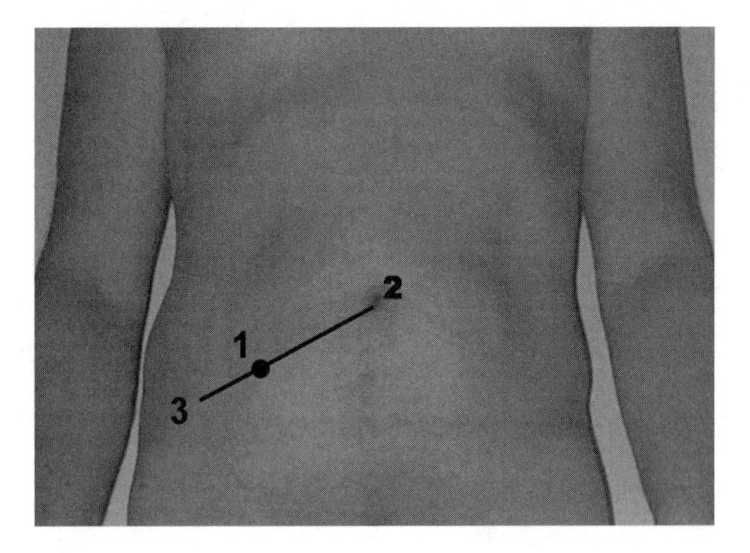

Figure 7.1

3. *Interventions:* anticipate orders to: give patient nothing by mouth (NPO), administer fluids intravenously, prepare a complete blood count, arrange for an abdominal CT scan, give antibiotics, and prepare for surgery.
   - A patient sent to surgery should be wearing only a gown. *No body jewelry in unusual places, no hearing aids, no dentures, no hairpins, no socks, no underwear—just a patient gown.*

*Notes:*____________________________________

____

____

Pancreatitis

This is the result of an increase in pancreatic enzymes. Whether it is caused by overproduction or obstruction, the enzymes erode or eat away the pancreatic tissues. Pancreatitis can spread to the liver, diaphragm, lungs, and other organs. It is basically the pancreas in self-destruct or autodigestion mode.

1. *Causes:* alcohol abuse; gallstones; infections; injury; autoimmune disorder; and drug toxicity. Contributing factors include smoking; stress; and crash dieting or binge eating.
2. *Signs and symptoms:* midepigastric abdominal pain radiating to the back; diminished bowel sounds; nausea and vomiting; abdominal distention; fever higher than 102°; jaundice if gallstones; weight loss; frothy and foul-smelling stools; dark urine; and altered blood sugar.

3. *Interventions:* anticipate orders to: administer fluids intravenously, monitor serum amylase, serum lipase, and blood glucose level, use nasogastric tube for decompression, administer nothing by mouth, give medications (antacids, anticholinergics, histamine receptor agonists, insulin, analgesics/narcotics), prevent and treat infections, prepare for possible surgery, and instruct patient on diet (low-fat diet, no caffeine, and no alcohol).
   - Normal serum amylase level? 25 to 125 U/L
   - The patient who is actively vomiting cannot drink water before seeing the emergency room provider *in case the patient ends up going to surgery.*

Notes: ____

____

____

Cholecystitis

Cholecystitis is an inflammation of the gallbladder.

1. *Causes:* gallstones; obstruction; or acute inflammation.
2. *Signs and symptoms:* right upper quadrant abdominal pain radiating to back or right shoulder that becomes worse after eating fatty foods; low-grade fever; clay-colored stool; nausea and vomiting; anorexia; flatulence; possible jaundice; fat intolerance; and Murphy's sign.
3. *Interventions:* anticipate orders to: arrange for gallbladder ultrasound, administer fluids intravenously, give medica-

tions (pain medications, sedatives for smooth muscle relaxation, antiemetics for nausea and vomiting), and use nasogastric tube for gastric decompression.

- *Morphine sulfate should be avoided.* It can cause gallbladder spasms.
- *Murphy's sign* is an increased sharp right upper quad abdominal pain that occurs during inspiration when palpating the patient's gallbladder and asking the patient to take a deep breath.
- To palpate the gallbladder, press the fingers under the right anterior rib cage.

Notes: ____

____

____

GI Bleeding

GI bleeding can be classified as upper or lower. Patients with gastrointestinal bleeding have a distinct odor. Once you have learned it, you can smell a patient with GI bleeding a mile away!

Upper gastrointestinal bleeding

1. *Causes:* esophageal varices; peptic ulcer; stomach cancer; alcohol abuse; and trauma.
2. *Signs and symptoms:* nausea and vomiting; blood that is bright red to coffeeground color; and black tarry stools or dark red rectal bleeding.

3. *Interventions:* anticipate orders to: start a 18- or 16-gauge intravenous access, prepare a complete blood count and coagulation studies, arrange for abdominal CT scan, use nasogastric tube, assess guaiac gastric contents and stool, administer fluids intravenously, give histamine antagonists, test blood for type and cross match, and prepare for possible blood transfusion.

Lower gastrointestinal bleeding

1. *Causes:* internal or external hemorrhoids; constipation; polyps; diverticulitis; colon cancer; and irritable bowel syndrome.
2. *Signs and symptoms:* bright red rectal bleeding.
3. *Interventions:* anticipate orders to: open large-bore intravenous access, prepare a complete blood count and coagulation studies, arrange for abdominal CT scan, insert nasogastric tube, assess guaiac gastric contents and stool, administer fluids intravenously, test blood for type and cross match, and prepare for possible blood transfusion.

Fast facts in a nutshell

- Ulcerative colitis and Crohn's Disease are inflammatory disorders of the colon and rectal mucosal lining. They can cause diffuse rectal bleeding.
- Pepto-Bismol, iron, and charcoal result in dark/black stools similar to upper gastrointestinal bleeding.

Question: Your patient arrives with history of alcohol abuse and cirrhosis. He is vomiting copious amounts of bright red blood. Vital signs are as follows: Blood pressue of 82/56, pulse of 144, respirations of 36, and temp of 99.8. What do you do first?
Answer: *suction blood from the airway (remember ABCs first).*

*Notes:*____

Fast facts in a nutshell: summary

Gastrointestinal emergencies are daily events in the emergency room. You should now be able to differentiate the various types of gastrointestinal emergencies. Be sure to assess, reassess, and document these patients carefully. Abdominal pain may involve a serious problem.

Chapter 8

Genitourinary Emergencies

INTRODUCTION

Genitourinary emergencies are routinely seen and treated in the emergency room. Most of the time they are minor problems that can be treated with medications. ***However, genitourinary problems, such as testicular torsion, can result in loss of life or limb if untreated.*** *This chapter will guide you through the genital and urinary problems commonly faced in the emergency room. After reviewing this chapter, you will understand the causes, manifestations, and interventions for common genitourinary emergencies.*

During this part of your orientation, locate and become familiar with:

1. Different types of Foley and straight catheters.
2. Bladder irrigation systems.

DIAGNOSES

Urinary Tract Infection

This is a bacterial infection of the bladder and urethra.

1. *Causes:* Because of their anatomy, UTIs are more common in women than in men. Other contributing factors are holding your urine, not drinking enough water, intercourse, and pH imbalances.
2. *Signs and symptoms:* painful urination (dysuria), hematuria, frequency, urgency, cloudy urine, foul-smelling urine, fever, and abdominal pain.
3. *Interventions:* obtain clean catch urine or catheter urine if vaginal bleeding is present, administer antibiotic as ordered, encourage fluids like cranberry juice and water, discourage caffeinated drinks, discourage bubble baths, encourage sitz baths, teach to wipe from front to back after toileting, and teach sexually active females to void and cleanse perineal area after intercourse. If administering phenazopyridine, teach that it will turn the urine orange and permanently stain underwear.

Notes: ____

____

____

Pyelonephritis

This is a bacterial infection of the kidney or renal pelvis.

1. *Causes:* pyelonephritis usually starts as a urinary tract infection in the urethra or bladder that travels all the way up to the kidneys.
2. *Signs and symptoms:* flank pain, painful urination (dysuria), hematuria, frequency, urgency, cloudy urine, foul-smelling urine, fever, chills, and nausea and vomiting.
   - Chronic pyelonephritis (renal failure): urine output less than 30 ml/hr (oliguria), elevated blood urea nitrogen and creatinine, hypertension, rapid weight gain, and altered loss of consciousness.
   - Urinalysis will reveal elevated white blood cell counts, elevated red blood cell counts, and bacteria.
3. *Interventions:* obtain clean catch urine or catheter urine if vaginal bleeding is present, intravenous fluids, and antibiotic/antipyretics/antiemetics as ordered, encourage fluids like cranberry juice and water, discourage caffeinated drinks, discourage bubble baths, encourage sitz baths and bed rest, teach females to wipe from front to back after toileting, and teach sexually active females to void and cleanse perineal area before and after intercourse.

*Notes:*____

____

____

Renal Calculi

Renal calculi are stones of various sizes along the urinary tract that are commonly known as kidney stones. This pain is equal to that experienced during childbirth!

1. *Causes:* kidney stones are usually made of calcium or uric acid salt deposits, possibly resulting from urine that is too alkaline or too acidic.
2. *Signs and symptoms:* SEVERE flank pain radiating to the groin, NV, hematuria, oliguria, pallor, diaphoresis, low-grade fever, and guarding.
3. *Interventions:* anticipate orders to: obtain clean catch or catheter urine if vaginal bleeding is present, start intravenous line, administer analgesics (intravenous Toradol) and evaluate for effectiveness, instruct to strain all urine, and prepare for CT scan of abdomen/pelvis without contrast. Don't forget to send patient home with a urine strainer.

*Notes:*______________________________________

____

____

Epididymitis

Epididymitis is an intrascrotal infection.

1. *Causes:* sexually transmitted diseases or urinary tract infections.

2. *Signs and symptoms:* penile discharge, bacteria in urinalysis, gradual scrotum pain, fever, epididymis swelling, and chills.
3. *Interventions:* anticipate orders for: ice pack to the scrotum, Gonorrhea and Chlamydia (G & C) culture, antibiotics, and instruct to abstain from sexual intercourse until follow-up repeat negative culture.

Fast facts in a nutshell

When preparing ceftriaxone (Rocephin) intramuscular injection (IM), 1% lidocaine may be used as a diluent to decrease discomfort.

*Notes:*____

____

____

Testicular Torsion

This occurs when a testis spontaneously twists one or more times on the cord, leading to possible ischemia. The most common age group is 12 to 18 years old.

1. *Causes:* It is not always known, but it can be attributed to an anatomic abnormality known as the bell clapper deformity. This deformity allows the cords to twist more easily.

2. *Signs and symptoms:* acute severe testicular pain radiating to groin or abdomen, nausea and vomiting, and elevated/swollen/tender testes.
3. *Interventions:* anticipate orders for: IV crystalloid fluids and analgesics, ice packs, testicular ultrasound; prepare for manual reduction of the torsion, or prepare for surgery as indicated.

*Notes:*____

____

____

Priapism

Priapism is a prolonged painful penile erection lasting longer than 4 to 6 hours.

1. *Common causes:* spinal cord injury, leukemia, sickle cell disease, psychotropic drugs, multiple sclerosis, prolonged sexual stimulation, penile tumor, urethral tumor, anticoagulant therapy, and impotence treatments.
2. *Signs and symptoms:* prolonged painful penile erection for more than 4 to 6 hours.
3. *Treatments:* anticipate treatment of underlying causes by provider that may include: observation of patient, ice packs, penile or groin pressure, intracavernous injections (with drugs like epinephrine, norepinephrine, ephedrine), needle aspiration, or surgery.

Fast facts in a nutshell

Question: How do you treat a 19-year-old male who arrives at the emergency room stating that his penis is stuck in his pants zipper?
Answer: *Cut it off. Not the penis, the zipper! Control bleeding and provide ice packs.*

Fast facts in a nutshell: summary

Although most genitourinary emergencies can be treated with medications, some can be life-threatening. You should now understand some of the most frequent problems that bring patients to the emergency room and how to treat them promptly and effectively.

Chapter 9

Geriatric Emergencies

INTRODUCTION

As the baby boomer generation ages, we can anticipate an even higher volume of ER patients. ***The normal physiological changes of the aging process leave patients more vulnerable to illness, injuries, and complications.*** *Several important body systems also slow down. Many geriatric patients have decreased renal function, decreased circulation, thinner skin, weaker bones, decreased hearing, decreased gastric motility, and visual impairments. It is always important to take these age-related changes into consideration when caring for older patients. As you review this chapter, you will learn some of the most common geriatric emergencies and how to handle them.*

During this part of your orientation, locate and become familiar with:

1. Assistive walking devices (e.g., canes, walkers).
2. Adult Protective Services and Social Services.

3. Facility policy for reporting elder abuse.
4. Denture containers.
5. Fall risk assessments and precautions.

DIAGNOSES

Fast facts in a nutshell

- Normal physiological changes leave older patients more vulnerable to illness, injuries, and complications.
- Geriatric patients may have decreased renal function, decreased circulation, thinner skin, weaker bones, decreased hearing, decreased gastric motility, and visual impairments.

Elder Abuse

Elder abuse can take several different forms, including physical, sexual, financial, and psychological; it can also include neglect. Abuse is physical harm, pain, or mental anguish; neglect is the failure to provide services or goods needed to prevent physical harm and mental anguish. Elder abuse is an international problem that can be difficult to detect. Females are more commonly abused than males. *You must report all suspected abuse!*

1. *Causes:* Not always known. Elder abuse can occur in any socioeconomic group. Lack of resources and stressed or burned-out caregivers can contribute to the problem.
2. *Signs and symptoms:* Conflicting stories describing how an injury occurred; patient not given an opportunity to speak; time lapse between injury and presentation to the emergency room; disinterested caregiver; history of similar injuries; hand marks; bite marks; multiple bruises; multiple fractures in various healing stages; altered ambulation from sexual assault; malnourishment; dehydration; poor hygiene; withdrawal; and agitation.
3. *Interventions:* treat injuries and illness; *accurately document* and photograph injuries or neglect per policy; ascertain if report needs to be filed; notify social services as soon as possible; obtain supportive services through community referrals; consider hospitalization to assure patient safety; and refer to *Adult Protective Services.*

*Notes:*____

Falls

Many geriatric injuries or illnesses are associated with falls. Complications often include soft tissue injuries, hip fractures, Colles' fracture (wrist), subdural hematoma, and hot water burns from falls in the bathtub. First, assess the reason for the fall. Were there any symptoms prior to the fall (e.g., dizziness, chest pain, loss of consciousness)? What was the activity during fall? the location? Are there any witnesses? Any history of falls or alcohol intake? Finally, assess if the patient fell at ground level. If not, how many feet did the patient fall?

1. *Causes:* can be attributed to impaired vision, gait, and balance.
2. *Signs and symptoms:* depends on the fall and injuries.
3. *Interventions:* nothing by mouth; consider cervical injury and immobilization (rest, ice, splint, and elevate injury); clean and apply sterile dressing to wounds; assess pain; administer pain medications as ordered; arrange neurological exams; monitor extremity movement; and check circulation.

*Notes:*____

____

____

Syncope

Syncope is transient loss of consciousness with a spontaneous recovery.

1. *Causes:* Identifying the cause may prove to be more valuable than treating the sustained injuries. Assess patient's activity just before the syncopal event.

   a. Temporary, abrupt decrease in cardiac output due to aortic stenosis, mitral valve disease, cardiomyopathy, dysrhythmias, and sick sinus syndrome.
   b. Volume depletion due to hemorrhage/anemia, diuresis, dehydration, and third-space fluid shift.
   c. Hypersensitive carotid sinus due to neck turning, constrictive collars, and drugs (digitalis, propranolol hydrochloride, alpha-methyldopa).
   d. Vasovagal response with hypotension due to cough, defecation, or urination.
   e. Hypoglycemia or hypoxia.
2. *Signs and symptoms:* dizziness; chest pain; dyspnea; weakness; confusion; loss of consciousness; witnesses to the fall; and previous history.
3. *Interventions:* anticipate orders to: obtain serum glucose or complete basic metabolic panel, administer 2 liters of oxygen through nasal cannula, check pulse oxygen, perform electrocardiogram, and check *orthostatic vital signs.*
   - If due to hypoglycemia, treat intravenously with D_{50} (1 amp) or give oral or intramuscular injection of glucose. Then feed patient once he or she is alert and oriented to person, place and time.

*Notes:*____

____

____

Dehydration

Dehydration is a lack of required serum fluid levels. Elderly patients are more prone to dehyration because of normal physiological changes.

1. *Causes:* altered sense of thirst; decrease in total body fluid; decreased kidney function; and decreased effectiveness of antidiuretic hormone, which helps conserve water.
2. *Signs and symptoms:* confusion; seizure; dry oral mucosa; dry skin; hyperthermia; weak rapid pulse; orthostatic hypotension; altered respiration; concentrated urine; and decreased urine output.
3. *Interventions:* anticipate orders to: administer fluids intravenously or by mouth, assess mental status, check orthostatic vital signs, and measure intake and output.

Notes: ____

____

____

Dementia

Dementia is age-related chronic mental impairment that may be the normal mental status for your patient. However, if the patient's symptoms in the emergency room are a new onset, the patient needs to be assessed for other causes, such as confusion due to electrolyte imbalance, dehydration, infection, and stroke. This assessment requires input from caregivers.

1. *Causes:* Unknown but may be attributed to physiological changes in the brain that occur with age.
2. *Signs and symptoms:* alert with impaired orientation; impaired recent memory; impoverished thinking; difficulty finding words; confused speech; and poor sleep.
3. *Interventions:* provide safe environment; put bed in low locked position; monitor patient closely (place close to nurses station); and assess for any new causes of confusion.
   - Common cause of confusion in elderly is *pneumonia* or *urinary tract infection.*

*Notes:*____

____

____

Alzheimer's Disease

Alzheimer's disease is chronic and progressive degenerative dementia that has no treatment or cure.

1. *Causes:* Unknown.
2. *Signs and symptoms:* forgetfulness; memory loss; paranoia; delusions; irritability; depression; aphasia; apraxia; and history of progressive deteriorating mental functioning.

3. *Interventions:* prevent patient from injuring self or others; provide supervised safe environment with minimal stimulation; give short explanations and simple instructions; involve supportive services (social services); and provide health care resources and community referrals.

*Notes:*___

___

___

Pneumonia

Pneumonia is a bacterial, viral, or fungal infection below the bronchi resulting in inflammation of lung parenchyma.

1. *Causes:* bacterial, viral, or fungal lung infection. Contributing factors include a weak immune system; general debilitated condition; decreased mobility; chronic cardiac disease; chronic pulmonary disease; weak cough reflex; aspiration; late diagnosis; and diabetes are all contributing factors.
2. *Signs and symptoms:* confusion; change in normal activity; anorexia; tachypnea; dyspnea; fever or subnormal temperature; dehydration; productive or nonproductive cough; chills; weakness; chest pain; nausea and vomiting; abdominal distention; diaphoresis; cyanosis; and diminished lung sounds or crackles.
3. *Interventions:* anticipate orders for: chest X-ray, a complete blood count, blood cultures, arterial blood gases. Start in-

travenous access, maintain bed rest, and give fluids intravenously, along with oxygen and antibiotics as ordered.

*Notes:*____

____

____

Urosepsis

Urosepsis is an infection caused by urinary tract infection that is more common in women than in men. In general, urinary infections are the most common bacterial infections in the elderly. Urosepsis may lead to septic shock.

1. *Causes:* Predisposing factors include an indwelling catheter and kidney stones.
2. *Signs and symptoms:* confusion; lethargy; altered mental status; tachycardia; tachypnea; fever or subnormal temperature; urinary frequency; urinary urgency; incontinence; nausea and vomiting; abdominal tenderness; and hypotension.
3. *Interventions:* anticipate orders to: obtain urinalysis (UA), administer fluids and antibiotics intravenously, and monitor urinary output.

*Notes:*____

____

____

Fast facts in a nutshell: summary

You now have a better understanding of the diseases most commonly associated with elderly patients in the ER. Age-related physiological changes in elderly patients will affect their condition and can lead to complications. Be sure to assess and document these patients carefully. Obtain histories from them and their caregivers, when available. Caring for elderly patients can be a blessing. Often they are more appreciative than younger patients.

Chapter 10

Infectious Disease Emergencies

INTRODUCTION

Infectious diseases are common emergencies that must not be taken lightly. Usually, it is the triage nurse who is first exposed to the unknown case of tuberculosis (TB) or meningitis. Most infectious disease patients don't know what is wrong with them when they come to the emergency room. Your facility should have a triage screening to alert the staff for infectious disease risks. If the triage screening is positive, you must follow your facilities protocol; this usually requires some sort of mask and isolation. The best advice I can give you is assess your patients ***carefully*** *and* ***wash your hands, wash your hands, wash your hands****! Most ER nurses frequently catch more colds and flus in their first year, so be careful. This chapter will educate you on the different types of infectious diseases and how to handle them.*

Fast facts in a nutshell

- Always practice Universal/Standard Precautions

During this part of your orientation, locate and become familiar with:

1. Wound cultures.
2. Lumbar puncture supplies, specimens, and procedures.
3. Contact, respiratory, and reverse isolation policies.
4. Personal protective equipment.
5. Incision and drainage supplies.
6. Triage screening for infectious diseases.
7. Policy for reporting disease to infection control personnel.

DIAGNOSES

Meningitis

Meningitis is a bacterial, viral, or fungal infection of the meninges, which are membrane coverings of the brain.

1. *Causes:* It usually starts as a sinus infection that spreads to the meninges.
2. *Signs and symptoms:* "the worst headache of my life"; stiff neck (nuchal rigidity); and high fever. Infants may be febrile; irritable; crying; have bulging fontanels; and have a poor appetite.

a. Kernig's sign is indicative of meningitis (low back/posterior thigh pain with hip flexion and gradual knee extension).

3. *Interventions:* place patient on droplet or airborne precautions during triage until test results return negative. Anticipate following orders: acetaminophen/ibuprofen for fever, monitor vital signs, prepare a complete blood count and blood culture, and prepare for lumbar puncture.
   - Bacterial meningitis reveals an elevated white blood cell (WBC) count greater than 1000 cells per mm^3 and low glucose in the cerebral spinal fluid. It is more serious and requires antibiotics like rifampin. Teach the patient that rifampin is an antibiotic that turns urine and tears orange.
   - Viral meningitis reveals mildly elevated white blood cell (WBC) count of 100–1000 cells per mm^3 or greater and normal glucose in the cerebral spinal fluid. It may require antiviral medication, but usually resolves on its own.

Fast facts in a nutshell

Providers will tell you positioning is key for obtaining a good lumbar puncture. For better positioning during a sitting lumbar puncture, place a step stool under the patient's feet. It brings the knees closer to the chest.

Notes: ______________________________________

____

____

HIV/AIDS

The human immunodeficiency virus (HIV) is a virus that attacks the immune system, allowing other pathogens to invade the body. Acquired immunodeficiency syndrome (AIDS) is a chronic, life-threatening condition caused by HIV. In the emergency room, we are to treat the acute complication of AIDS.

1. *Causes:* Contamination by the human immunodeficiency virus (HIV) through blood or body fluid exchange.
2. *Signs and symptoms:* early manifestations are similar to cold and flu symptoms. Later symptoms include weight loss; fever; shortness of breath; mouth ulcers; cough; sores that won't heal; and swollen lymph nodes.
   - Abnormally low CD4 lymphocyte count may be present.
   - Common opportunistic infections include bacterial pneumonia; tuberculosis; herpes; human papillomavirus; thrush; cryptococcal meningitis; Pneumocystis carinii pneumonia; Kaposi's sarcoma; and non-Hodgkin's lymphoma.
3. *Interventions:* anticipate orders to: treat opportunistic infections, maintain appropriate isolation depending on complications, monitor vital signs, administer acetaminophen for fever, prepare a complete blood count, perform HIV testing (ELISA and western blot tests) if unknown case, request chest X-ray (CXR), culture wounds, and obtain intravenous access.

Fast facts in a nutshell

We do not perform routine HIV testing in the emergency room because we can not provide follow-up care. Your local Health Department can provide routine HIV testing.

Hepatitis

Hepatitis is an inflammation or infection of the liver.

1. *Causes:* alcohol abuse; overdose of medications; and presence of hepatitis A virus, hepatitis B virus, or hepatitis C virus.
2. *Signs and symptoms:* ascites; jaundice; elevated liver enzymes; right upper quadrant abdominal pain; and nausea and vomiting. The patient often looks like Big Bird—yellow all over with a big round belly.
3. *Interventions:* anticipate orders to: medicate for pain, nausea, and vomiting, complete a basic metabolic panel, perform a liver function test and coagulation studies, check for abnormal bleeding, and educate the patient to stop any alcohol consumption or use of Tylenol.

Notes: ______________________________

____

____

Cellulitis/Abscess/MRSA

Abscesses are pockets of skin infection that look like giant pimples from the size of a marble to a golf ball or larger. Diabetic patients are at higher risk for cellulitis and poor healing.

1. *Causes:* Most abscesses are caused from methicillin-resistant Staphylococcus aureus (MRSA). Others may come from other types of bacteria, clogged hair follicles, or clogged pores.
2. *Signs and symptoms:* pain; redness and warmth to affected area; proximal red streaks; pus; and/or fever.
3. *Interventions:* anticipate orders to: prepare patient for possible incision and drainage of abscess; if appropriate, pack the wound, bandage the wound, administer antibiotics and warm compresses. *Educate the patient on how to prevent the spread of MRSA (wash hands and bleach everything). MRSA lives dormant under fingernails and in nostrils. This is why your mom said not to pick your nose! Providers may prescribe antibiotic ointment to apply inside nostrils.

Notes: ____

____

____

Febrile Neutropenia

A febrile neutropenic patient is immunocompromised with a fever or a possible infection.

1. *Causes:* These are usually patients receiving chemotherapy. For them, a low-grade fever, say 99.9°, is of concern because their immune systems are too weak to handle it.
2. *Signs and symptoms:* fever and possibly cold- or flu-like symptoms.
3. *Interventions:* reverse isolation with neutropenic precautions. During triage or in waiting room, provide patient with a mask for his or her own protection until placed in isolation room. Monitor vital signs; anticipate orders to: administer acetaminophen or ibuprofen (for fever) and antibiotics, prepare a complete blood count, obtain an intravenous access, and prepare for possible admission.

*Notes:*____

____

____

Tick-Borne Illnesses

These are infectious diseases caused by ticks.

Lyme Disease: a Borrelia burgdorferi bacterial infection. See Figure 10.1.

1. *Causes:* Usually spread by deer ticks.
2. *Signs and symptoms:* vary by individual, but commonly include a "bull's-eye" rash at site of tick bite; flu-like symptoms; joint pain; fatigue; and neurologic problems.
3. *Interventions:* remove all ticks and administer antibiotics (e.g., doxycycline or amoxicillin) as ordered.

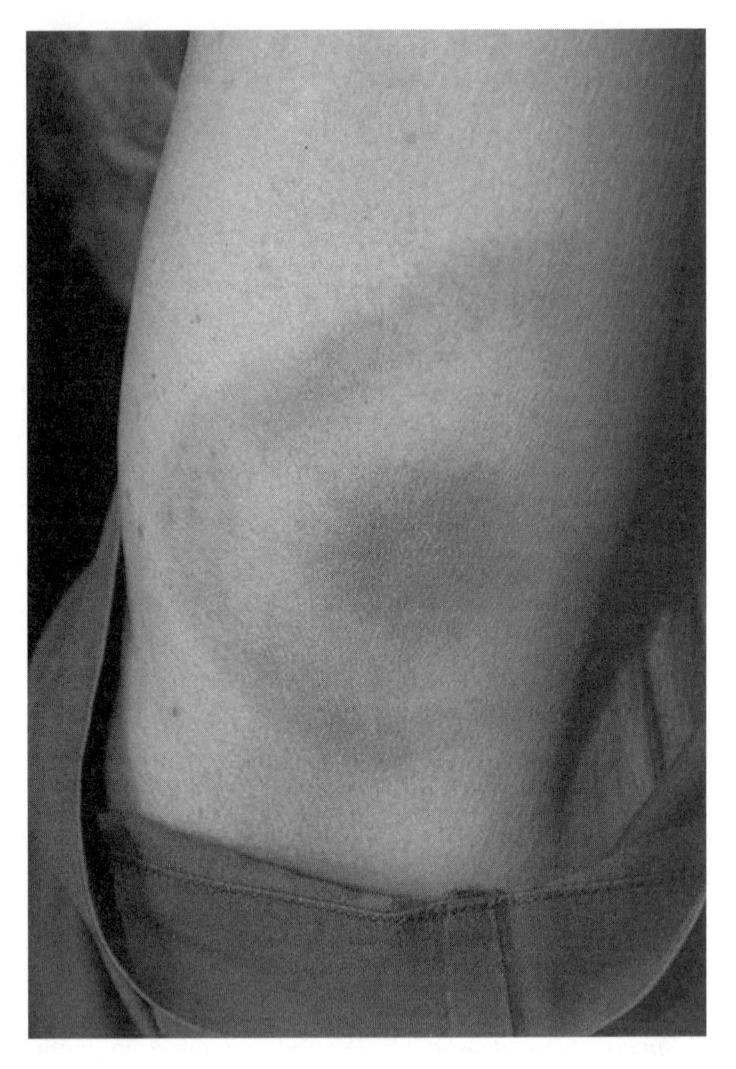

Figure 10.1

Rocky Mountain spotted fever: a bacterial infection transmitted by ticks.

1. *Causes:* bite from tick contaminated with bacteria.
2. *Signs and symptoms:* high fever; recent tick bite 2 to 14 days earlier; sore throat; headache; nausea and vomiting; fatigue; and red spotted rash.
3. *Interventions:* remove all ticks and administer antibiotics (e.g., doxycycline or tetracycline) as ordered.

Fast facts in a nutshell

- For easy tick removal, dab some Vaseline to area before pulling on the head portion.
- To remove a tick, steadily pull from the head.

*Notes:*____

____

____

Toxic Shock Syndrome

Toxic shock syndrome is a life-threatening Staphylococcus aureus or group A Beta-hemolytic Strep bacterial infection.

1. *Causes:* Commonly occurs with the use of tampons vaginally or nasally. The toxins released from these two bacteria

can cause the patient to go into septic shock *very rapidly*—sometimes right before your eyes.

2. *Signs and symptoms:* similar to septic shock but faster. Includes sudden high fever; hypotension; headache; confusion; tachycardia; nausea, vomiting, and diarrhea; sunburn-like rash; fatigue; and seizures.
3. *Interventions:* You must work rapidly. Monitor vital signs; anticipate orders to: insert a large-bore intravenous access for administration of intravenous isotonic fluid bolus and, as soon as possible, antibiotics, place in modified Trendelenburg position for hypotension, prepare a complete blood count, take blood cultures, remove any foreign body to any body cavity and get a wound culture (if source is vaginal, prepare for pelvic exam with cultures), give norepinephrine or dopamine for hypotension, and prepare for possible intensive care unit admission.
   - If the patient is stable, try to obtain blood cultures before giving antibiotics. If unstable, give the antibiotics now!*

Notes: ____

____

____

Tuberculosis

In its *active phase,* tuberculosis is a life-threatening bacterial infection that commonly attacks the lungs but can attack other organs as well.

1. *Causes:* It is spread via droplet, so negative pressure respiratory isolation is necessary. In its dormant stage, it is not contagious, and patient is asymptomatic.
2. *Signs and symptoms:* the patient can be asymptomatic or have cough lasting several weeks; coughing up blood; fever; night sweats; and fatigue.
3. *Interventions:* screen patients for tuberculosis in triage and provide mask to suspected patients. Then place the patient in room on respiratory isolation. Anticipate orders to: obtain intravenous access, request a chest X-ray, obtain a complete blood count, administer antibiotics (e.g., isoniazid and rifampin), and prepare for possible admission. Instruct family members and caregivers to get tuberculosis testing.

Fast facts in a nutshell

Question: What drug besides phenazopyridine (Pyridium) makes your urine orange?
Answer: *rifampin*

*Notes:*____

____

____

Fast facts in a nutshell: summary

Most emergency rooms don't allow new graduate nurses to triage until proper training and experience is achieved. This is partly because the triage nurses are the front line when it comes to exposure to infectious diseases. Therefore, it is crucial to thoroughly screen all patients that come through triage for infectious diseases. If an infectious disease is suspected, proper isolation must be implemented. Make sure you become familiar with your facility's isolation protocols and equipment and know how to use it. This information may seem a bit scary at first, but look around you. There are emergency room nurses who have been doing this for decades! The key is good hand washing, universal precautions, triage screening, and proper isolation.

Chapter 11

Mental Health Emergencies

INTRODUCTION

I have to admit, mental health emergencies are not everyone's favorite topic. Just in the last 10 years, ***the way we deal with mental health emergencies has changed dramatically.*** *For instance, nurses used to automatically put suicidal patients in seclusion "for their own protection" and used restraints more freely. Most mentally healthy people would go crazy under such conditions. We can all empathize; everyone experiences anxiety, stress, anger, and depression in their lives, but some people become suicidal, violent, or psychotic. Mental health patients may be difficult to treat at times, particularly when they engage in disruptive behavior. At times security, seclusion, and restraints may be necessary for short periods of time.* ***Your priority must always be to maintain safety for yourself, your staff members, your patient, and other patients.*** *However, you will find that most mental health patients respond better if you listen, respect their personal space, and educate them on all procedures clearly and early on.*

During this part of your orientation, locate and become familiar with:

1. Your state's and facility's seclusion and restraint policies.
2. Restrain-and-seclusion forms.
3. Legal suicidal intent documents.
4. Transfer policies to mental health facilities.
5. Local mental health counselors and facilities.
6. Your facility's security and its codes.
7. Drugs: lorazepam (Ativan) and haloperidol (Haldol).

DIAGNOSES

Anxiety

Anxiety is a vague feeling of apprehension, tension, and uneasiness that can be divided into four levels: mild, moderate, severe, and panic.

1. *Causes:* Usually some sort of stressor, but it varies with the individual and his or her circumstances.
2. *Signs and symptoms by level*
   a. *Mild:* minimal muscle tension; normal vital signs; constricted normal pupils; random controlled thoughts; and appearance of calm.
   b. *Moderate:* normal to slightly elevated vital signs; tension; excited behavior; alertness; optimum state for problem solving and learning; attentive; and energized.
   c. *Severe:* flight-or-fight response; tachycardia; tachypnea; hypertension; diaphoretic; urinary urgency; diarrhea;

dry mouth; dilated pupils; difficulty in problem solving; feel overwhelmed; and decreased appetite.
   d. *Panic:* faint feeling or syncope from sympathetic nervous system release; pallor; hyperventilation; hypertension; pain; weakness; lack of coordination; choking or gasping sensation; chest pressure or lump in throat; helplessness; may become angry/combative/withdrawn, tearful; and shortness of breath.
3. *Interventions:* maintain calm and private environment; reduce stimulation; stay with the patient or have a support person stay; use simple repetitive communication; encourage verbalization of feelings; administer antianxiety/analgesic medications; evaluate effectiveness of medications; and teach relaxation/breathing techniques.

*Notes:*____

____

____

Posttraumatic Stress Disorder

The disorder is a reaction to overwhelmingly traumatic events.

1. *Causes:* a traumatic or overwhelming event.
2. *Signs and symptoms:* signs of anxiety or stress; recurring dreams or flashbacks; explosive anger; increased substance abuse; and feelings of guilt.
3. *Interventions:* assess suicidal/homicidal ideations; assess anxiety levels; provide therapeutic listening; avoid judg-

ment; and provide referrals for group or individual counseling.

*Notes:*____

____

____

Depression

Depresssion is a state of sadness that affects one mentally and physically. Short periods of depression following a specific event, such as divorce or death, are natural and resolve in time. However, clinical depression related to chemical or hormonal imbalances may require medication and therapy for a lifetime.

1. *Causes:* Vary by individual and circumstances. May be the natural result of a specific event, such as divorce or death. If, however, it is the result of hormonal or chemical imbalances, the condition may require prolonged treatment.
2. *Signs and symptoms:* sad mood; lack of interest in or pleasure from activities; insomnia or hypersomnia; fatigue; feeling of guilt or worthlessness; inability to think or concentrate; inability to make decisions; and suicidal ideation or attempt.
3. *Interventions:* assess suicide risk; discuss patient's emotional state; show interest and concern; and provide choices. Antidepressants are rarely administered in the emergency room, they are not usually effective for the first week or two.

Fast facts in a nutshell

- Tricyclics = amitriptyline (Elavil) and imipramine (Tofranil)
- Tricyclic antidepressants + alcohol = hypertensive crisis
- Monoamine Oxidase Inhibitors (MAOIs) + foods that ferment (yogurt, cheeses, sour cream) = hypertensive crisis

Fast facts in a nutshell

Question: Why don't we discharge patients with antidepressant prescriptions?
Answer: *These patients need psychiatric follow-up and probably will not go if they are able to receive medications in the emergency department.*

*Notes:*____

Suicide

Suicide is an intentional self-inflicted death. Suicidal actions include suicidal thoughts, threats, gestures, and/or attempts.

1. *Causes:* Vary by individual and circumstance. There are, however, common risk factors: male; age over 65; Caucasian; substance/physical /sexual/mental/emotional abuse; depression; family history of or prior suicide attempt; terminal or chronic illness; psychosis; lives alone; recent change/loss in life; and low self-esteem.
2. *Signs and symptoms:* previous suicide attempts; verbal statements of suicidal thoughts; giving away favorite items; writing a will; depressed mood; isolated; and withdrawn.
3. *Interventions:* engage in one-to-one observation; remove any potentially dangerous objects (dress in a gown and remove personal belongings); encourage verbal expression of feelings/thoughts; promote hope; obtain labs as ordered for medical clearance; and obtain mental health evaluation. Assessment questions are listed below.
   - Have you thought of harming yourself?
   - Are you thinking of harming yourself?
   - How would you do it?
   - Is this method accessible to you?
   - Do you hope to die or be rescued?
   - When are you planning on killing yourself?
   - What has kept you from killing yourself?
   - Who is available to help you?

Fast facts in a nutshell

- The 20-year-old suicidal male patient who describes to you how he is going to commit suicide is the most dangerous.

*Notes:*____

____

____

Violent or Aggressive Behavior

This is behavior that has harmed or may result in harm to the patient or others.

1. *Causes:* Many factors can trigger aggressive behavior, including alcohol, drugs, or long waiting times.
2. *Signs and symptoms:* loud/threatening speech; yelling profanities; bragging about past violence; demanding personality; pacing; acting tense; clenching fists; slamming/pushing/throwing objects; alcohol odor; or other unusual behavior.
3. *Interventions:* It's tough, but you have to stay calm; speak softly/slowly/clearly; respect patient's personal space; provide brief and honest facts; be an empathetic listener; encourage patient to verbalize feelings; provide "show-of-force" with security if needed; restrain as last resort; medicate as ordered and as necessary; and document all interventions and behaviors.
   - There are some people you cannot make happy no matter what you do. When you have tried everything listed above, tell the person you will find someone to help and calmly *walk away!* Then chart the person's behavior and your interventions. Notify your charge nurse or supervisor that you require assistance.

*Notes:*____________________________________

____

____

Psychosis

Psychosis is when a patient's reality is grossly impaired. It is commonly associated with schizophrenia.

1. *Causes:* Origin may be unknown, but the patient must be medically cleared. Some brain injuries and chemical imbalances can also cause psychosis.
2. *Signs and symptoms:* delusions; hallucinations; disorganized speech; paranoia; poverty of speech; and flat affect.
3. *Interventions:* reorient to reality; maintain calm professional manner; explain unseen noises/voices/activities clearly and simply; give Haldol as ordered; and respect patient's personal space.

Fast facts in a nutshell

- Do not touch a patient who is hallucinating.
- The drug of choice for acute psychotic behavior is haloperidol (Haldol) administered by injection or intravenously.

Notes: ____

____

____

Manic Behavior

Manic behavior is an elevated, unstable, or irritable mood. Bipolar disorder includes manic and depressive behaviors.

1. *Causes:* Bipolar disorder and drug use are common.
2. *Signs and symptoms:* euphoria; grandiosity; insomnia; flight of ideas; aggression; easily distracted; impulsive; increased motor activity; and very talkative. You can't get one word in with these patients.
3. *Interventions:* reduce stimuli; obtain urine drug screen and lithium level as ordered; reorient to reality; use "show of force" as needed with security for aggressive behavior; set limits on manipulative/negative behavior; restrain as needed for safety according to policy.

Fast facts in a nutshell

A manic patient is at risk for harming himself or others because of reckless behavior.

*Notes:*____

____

____

Fast facts in a nutshell: summary

You should now have a better understanding of mental health emergencies and how to handle them. From sad and suicidal patients to loud and schizophrenic patients wearing lampshades on their heads, you never know what kind of mental health challenge you will face next in the emergency room. Nevertheless, your mental health patients will respond better when you remain calm, speak concisely, respect personal space, and inform patients of upcoming procedures. There are important legal issues and patient rights regarding mental health emergencies. Document carefully and become familiar with your state's and facility's legal forms and policies regarding suicide, restraints, and seclusion. In addition, know how to get a hold of security personnel if you need them right away. You may find that mental health emergencies can be tough, sad, and rewarding.

Chapter 12

Neurological Emergencies

INTRODUCTION

The neurological system is a critical piece of the human puzzle. It is fascinating and fragile. There are many different forms of neurological emergencies. In the emergency room, you may see anything from head trauma with grand mal seizures to Bell's palsy. It is important to get a good history and neurological assessment on these patients. This chapter will help you learn the major neurological emergencies and how to handle them.

During this part of your orientation, become familiar with and locate:

1. Stroke protocol for your facility.
2. Neurological assessment tools (Glasgow Coma Scale).
3. Drugs to learn: heparin, warfarin (Coumadin), nitroglycerin, sodium nitroprusside (Nipride), phenytoin (Dilantin), diazepam (Valium), and lorazepam (Ativan).

PLAN FOR THE WORST, HOPE FOR THE BEST

I will never forget a patient who took me by surprise. He came in unconscious and postictal from a witnessed seizure with no history and no family. We were treating him for a routine seizure when he suddenly became hypertensive with multiple seizures, and we learned of his history of uncontrolled hypertension. He was having a massive hemorrhagic stroke—and not just a routine seizure! He needed a head CT scan superstat.

DIAGNOSES

Stroke (Cerebrovascular Accident)

A stroke is is an interruption of cerebral circulation, also known as a cerebrovascular accident (CVA). The three types of strokes are listed below, along with their causes, manifestations, and interventions.

Ischemic

1. *Causes:* clot; thrombus; embolus; compression; or spasm.
2. *Signs and symptoms:* usually occurs while sleeping. Symptoms, which vary depending on location, magnitude, and duration, include arm drift; pupil changes; paralysis; facial droop; weakness; nausea and vomiting; hearing loss; headache; altered mental status; aphasia; dysphasia; receptive aphasia; visual disturbances; vertigo; ataxia; symptoms of increased intracranial pressure; and seizure.

3. *Interventions:* follow hospital stroke protocol (usually 2–3 hour window from onset of symptoms to treatment); maintain patent airway; watch cardiac and blood pressure monitor; administer oxygen; order CT scan of the head; give antihypertensive medications if systolic blood pressure is greater than 220 and diastolic blood pressure is greater than 120 (don't lower blood pressure fast!); perform coagulation studies, electrocardiogram, and frequent neurological assessments; and give anticoagulants (e.g., heparin, warfarin [Coumadin], antiplatelet medication (e.g., aspirin), and thrombolytics (tissue plasminogen activator or TPA, urokinase, and streptokinase).

Hemorrhagic

1. *Causes:* rupture of cerebral blood vessel.
2. *Signs and symptoms:* often occur upon waking or shortly thereafter. Symptoms, which vary depending on location, magnitude, and duration, include arm drift; pupil changes; paralysis; facial droop; weakness; nausea and vomiting; hearing loss; headache; altered mental status; aphasia; dysphasia; receptive aphasia; visual disturbances; vertigo; ataxia; symptoms of increased intracranial pressure; and seizure.
3. *Interventions:* follow hospital stroke protocol (usually 2–3 hour window from onset of symptoms to treatment); maintain patent airway; watch cardiac and blood pressure monitor; administer oxygen; anticipate order for: CT scan of the head, antihypertensive medications if systolic blood pressure is greater than 220 and diastolic blood pressure is greater than 120 (don't lower blood pressure too fast!),

perform coagulation studies, electrocardiogram, and frequent neurological assessments. Consider surgical intervention. Prepare for operating room admission with neurosurgeon or transfer as ordered.

Transient Ischemic Attack: A ministroke, also known as a transient ischemic attack (TIA), is a temporary interruption of cerebral blood flow that resolves on its own.

1. *Causes:* temporary interruption of blood supply from a clot, spasm, or cerebral bleeding.
2. *Signs and symptoms:* Symptoms, which vary depending on location, magnitude, and duration, persist less than 24 hours without permanent neurological deficit. They include arm drift; pupil changes; paralysis; facial droop; weakness; nausea and vomiting; hearing loss; headache; altered mental status; aphasia; dysphasia; receptive aphasia; visual disturbances; vertigo; ataxia; symptoms of increased intracranial pressure; and seizure.
3. *Interventions:* follow hospital stroke protocol (usually 2–3 hour window from onset of symptoms to treatment); maintain patent airway; watch cardiac and blood pressure monitor; administer oxygen; anticipate order for: CT scan of the head, antihypertensive medications if systolic blood pressure is greater than 220 and diastolic blood pressure is greater than 120 (don't lower BP too fast!), coagulation studies, electrocardiogram, and frequent neurological assessments, and prepare for admission.

Fast facts in a nutshell

Question: What do you give for warfarin (Coumadin) overdose?
Answer: *Vitamin K.*

Question: What do you give for heparin overdose?
Answer: *Protamine sulfate.*

Question: Patient states "it is the worst headache of his life," and he has nausea and vomiting; photosensitivity; hypertension; bradycardia; and aphasia. What is the most likely diagnosis?
Answer: *Ruptured cerebral aneurysm.*

Question: What are the guidelines for administering nitroprusside for hypertension?
Answer: *Protect from light; use provided covering. Average dose is 3 to 10 mcg/kg/min.*

Notes: ____________________

____

____

Seizures

A seizure is sudden interruption of electrical brain activity, followed by postictal state. Many different types are listed below, but the treatment is always the same.

1. *Causes:* Aside from febrile seizures, the cause is not always known. Underlying conditions include brain tumor, cerebral infarct, head trauma, medication overdose, and alcohol abuse.
2. *Signs and symptoms:*. Each type of seizure, with specific signs and symptoms, is listed below.
   a. *Generalized absence seizure (petit mal):* characterized by staring or eyelid fluttering for 5 to 10 seconds.
   b. *Tonic clonic (grand mal):* generalized stiffening of extremities, followed by jerking movements; sweating; frothing at the mouth; incontinence; and amnesia.
   c. *Partial (focal):* affect only part of the brain. Symptoms vary according to location of the seizure. It is usually accompanied by an aura. Focal seizures may be the result of underlying problems (e.g., trauma, tumor, or infarct).
   d. *Focal motor:* starts with focal jerking that may persist or may spread to the entire body (grand mal).
   e. *Febrile:* common in infants and young children with high fever.
   f. *Status epilepticus:* the seizure that never ends and is therefore an emergency! The patient keeps having one seizure after another so it looks like one long seizure. The patient with status epilepticus will have increased temperature, blood pressure, and pulse. The patient is at risk for hypoxic brain damage.
   g. *Pseudoseizures:* when the patient is faking a seizure. Yes, this does actually happen! Patient movements may be purposeful, but the patient is not postictal after a fake seizure. This type of seizure is usually preceded by emotional upset, generally lasts longer than a true seizure, and the patient shows stable vital signs.

- Arm Test: hold the patient's arm above his or her face, and let go. A truly unconscious patient will hit his or her face with the arm. The pseudoseizure patient will avoid hitting the face.
- Wave ammonia in front of the patient. If it is a pseudoseizure, the patient will suddenly be alert and oriented to person, place, and time.

3. *Interventions:* protect the patient from harm but do not restrain; protect airway; place in recovery position afterward; administer oxygen; anticipate order to: obtain an intravenous access, give medications (lorazepam, diazepam, and anticonvulsants), and reorient to reality after postictal state.

Fast facts in a nutshell

Question: How fast do you give phenytoin (Dilantin)?
Answer: *No faster than 50 mg/min using an in-line filter to avoid cardiac arrhythmias and cardiac arrest. In addition, phenytoin (Dilantin) commonly causes phlebitis. If it infiltrates, it causes tissue necrosis!*

Question: Does Dilantin treat petit mal seizures?
Answer: *No!*

Question: What intravenous solution can be mixed with Dilantin?
Answer: *Saline only (think Seizure, think Saline). Any other solution causes drug to crystallize.*

Question: What can be mixed with diazepam (Valium) administered intravenously?
Answer: *Absolutely nothing, not even saline, as it will turn chalky.*

*Notes:*____

Bell's Palsy

Bell's palsy is paralysis of cranial nerve VII (facial). It usually resolves in several weeks to months.

1. *Causes:* Unknown, but it is thought to be caused by a virus or immunodeficiency disorder.
2. *Signs and symptoms:* facial paralysis; headache; facial swelling; numbness; inability to close one eye; facial droop; and drooling.
3. *Interventions:* give medications (steroids, analgesics, artificial tears) as ordered and reassure the patient that he or she is not having a stroke.

*Notes:*____

Myasthenia Gravis

Myasthenia gravis is a neuromuscular disorder.

1. *Causes:* Thought to be caused by a myoneural junction defect.
2. *Signs and symptoms:* voluntary muscle weakness, especially of the face. Symptoms may improve with rest. Tensilon test is used to diagnose myasthenia gravis, as shown by the significant improvement of the patient after edrophonium is given intravenously.
3. *Interventions:* perform neurological assessments and give anticholinesterase drugs as ordered.

Fast facts in a nutshell

Question: What is the antidote for anticholinesterase toxicity?
Answer: *Atropine.*

*Notes:*____

____

____

Multiple Sclerosis

Multiple sclerosis is a chronic autoimmune disorder in which the body attacks its own myelin sheaths, thereby damaging nerve impulses. The damage affects muscle coordination, strength, sensation, and vision.

1. *Causes:* Unknown.
2. *Signs and symptoms:* diplopia; scotomas; tremor; blindness; weakness; fatigue; bladder/bowel incontinence; emotional instability; and paralysis.
3. *Interventions:* anticipate order to: administer diazepam, baclofen, and gabapentin to decrease spasms and tremors.

Notes: ____

____

____

Cluster Headache

A cluster headache is not one headache, but cycles of very painful headaches over 2 to 12 weeks.

1. *Causes:* Unknown but alcohol use can aggravate the headaches.
2. *Signs and symptoms:* Vary with individual, but usually include pain on one side of the face or eye; runny nose; and nausea and vomiting. Usually, the patient has one tearful, puffy, red eye.

3. *Interventions:* give pain medication, sumatriptan succinate (Imitrex) by subcutaneous injection, administer 100% oxygen via nonrebreather for 7 to 8 minutes and then rest.

Notes: ____

____

____

TABLE 12.1 Glasgow Coma Scale

Eye opening	Verbal response	Motor response
4 spontaneously	5 orientated	6 obeys commands
3 to speech	4 confused	5 localized to pain
2 to pain	3 inappropriate	4 withdraws to pain
1 none	2 incomprehensible	3 flexion to pain
	1 none	2 extension to pain
		1 none

Fast facts in a nutshell

- The Glasgow Coma Scale (Table 12.1) assesses impaired consciousness by evaluating a patient's eye movement, body movement, and verbal responses. A patient with no eye movement, body movement, or verbal response would score a three.

- Contraindications for lumbar puncture include taking warfarin (Coumadin); increased intracranial pressure; intracranial bleed; or infection of the lumbar puncture site.

Fast facts in a nutshell: summary

You now have a basic knowledge of neurological emergencies. You should be able to differentiate the various types and know how to treat them. Documenting a patient's complete history and neurological assessments is absolutely vital. Be familiar with your facility's neurological assessment tools, such as the Glasgow Coma Scale. Never underestimate your patient's symptoms. Sometimes a simple headache is the result of cerebral aneurysms or brain masses. Therefore concise assessments and rapid testing is key.

Chapter 13

OB/GYN Emergencies

INTRODUCTION

Obstetrical and gynecological emergencies occur regularly in the emergency room. As a nurse, you must be familiar and comfortable with the various types of OB/GYN emergencies. This chapter will guide you through the many common types of obstetrical and gynecological challenges you will face in the emergency room. When caring for these patients, be sure to always respect your patient's privacy by closing doors and curtains and providing blankets for covering up. Patients may be uncomfortable talking about obstetrical or gynecological matters. It is also true that some women are not well educated about their bodies. Some actually do deliver full-term babies in the emergency room without knowing they were pregnant. ***Thus, the nurse must be sure to document a full and accurate triage and secondary assessment to find the source of the patient's complaint.*** *You may have to ask a lot of questions to get the necessary patient history.*

During this part of your orientation, locate and become familiar with:

1. Precipitous delivery tray.
2. Pelvic examination equipment and specimen supplies.
3. Drugs to know: ceftriaxone (Rocephin), azithromycin (Zithromax), RhoGAM injection, and methotrexate.
4. Doppler for fetal heart tones.

DIAGNOSES

Endometriosis

Endometriosis is a painful menstrual cycle that occurs because endometrial tissue fragments are found outside the uterus.

1. *Causes:* the abnormal tissue fragments react to hormones and slough during menstruation, thereby causing pelvic pain.
2. *Signs and symptoms:* pelvic pain with menstruation; dysuria; irregular menstrual cycles; and abnormal uterine bleeding.
3. *Interventions:* as ordered, administer analgesic medication and evaluate effectiveness; bed rest; set up and assist in pelvic examination; refer patient to OB/GYN specialist.

Notes: ____

____

____

Bartholin's Cyst

Bartholin's cyst is an obstruction/abscess of the Bartholin gland. The Bartholin gland is responsible for vaginal secretions during sexual arousal.

1. *Causes:* STI causing a clogged or obstructed Bartholin gland.
2. *Signs and symptoms:* pain with intercourse and vaginal lump or abscess.
3. *Interventions:* anticipate orders to: administer analgesic/narcotic medications and assess effectiveness, prepare for incision and drainage, assist with Word catheter insertion, administer antibiotics, and teach patient about sitz baths.

*Notes:*____

____

____

Vaginitis

Vaginitis is a general term for an altered normal vaginal flora pH.

1. *Causes:* aquired immunodeficiency syndrome; allergic reaction; bacterial vaginosis; Trichomonas vaginitis; foreign object (e.g., old tampon); and yeast (Candida albicans) infection.
2. *Signs and symptoms:* red inflamed vaginal mucosa and abnormal vaginal discharge (see Table 13.1).

TABLE 13.1

Bacterial vaginosis	Candida albicans
Gray–white, thin, fish odor vaginal discharge Give metronidazole or clindamycin by mouth	White, curd cheese-like vaginal discharge Medications fluconazole (Diflucan) by mouth or miconazole intravaginally

3. *Interventions:* prepare for pelvic exam with culture specimen collection; as ordered, administer medication according to offending organism, pelvic rest, and patient teaching.

*Notes:*____

Pelvic Inflammatory Disease

Pelvic infammatory disease is a vaginal bacterial infection that ascends into and beyond the cervix.

1. *Causes:* Usually starts as a vaginal bacterial infection that spreads into and beyond the cervix.

2. *Signs and symptoms:* fever; lower abdominal pain with rebound tenderness; irregular menstrual cycle; foul-odor vaginal discharge; cervical inflammation; "the PID shuffle," shuffling gait due to pain; elevated white blood cell count; and severe pain on pelvic examination.
3. *Interventions:* prepare cultures for pelvic exam; bed rest; anticipate orders to: administer analgesic/narcotic pain medications, evaluate pain medication effectiveness, give fluids intravenously or by mouth, administer antibiotics, and teach patient about pelvic rest.

Fast facts in a nutshell

Question: Which microorganism is the most common cause of PID?
Answer: *Neisseria gonorrhea*

Notes: ______________________________

____

____

Spontaneous Abortion (Miscarriage)

Miscarriage occurs before the 20th week of gestation. Table 13.2 shows the various types of miscarriages: complete, incomplete, threatened, inevitable, septic, and missed.

TABLE 13.2 Types of Miscarriages

Threatened	Complete	Incomplete or Inevitable	Septic	Missed
Symptoms				
Slight vaginal bleeding; mild uterine cramps; and closed cervical opening; extrauterine pregnancy on ultrasound, fetal heart tones.	Slight vaginal bleeding; mild uterine cramps; closed cervical opening; and no intrauterine pregnancy on ultrasound.	Severe vaginal bleeding and clots; moderate uterine cramps; open cervical opening; and ruptured amniotic membranes.	Foul vaginal discharge and bleeding; uterine cramps; fever; and open cervical opening.	Slight vaginal bleeding; closed cervical opening; and no fetal heart beat or intrauterine products of conception noted on ultrasound.

Interventions

Pelvic exam and pelvic ultrasound; RhoGAM injection if Rh is negative; bed rest; pelvic rest;* and Ob/Gyn doctor follow-up.	Pelvic exam and pelvic ultrasound; RhoGAM injection if Rh is negative; bed rest; pelvic rest;* and Ob/Gyn doctor follow-up.	Pelvic exam and pelvic ultrasound; RhoGAM injection if Rh is negative; bed rest; pelvic rest;* and Ob/Gyn follow-up.	Pelvic exam and pelvic ultrasound; blood cultures; intravenous access; antibiotics; recheck temperature and vital signs; give RhoGAM injection if Rh is negative; bed rest; pelvic rest;* and Ob/Gyn doctor follow-up.	Pelvic exam and pelvic ultrasound; coagulation studies; bed rest; pelvic rest;* Ob/Gyn doctor follow-up; and prepare for surgical intervention.

* Pelvic rest means no sexual intercourse and no tampons; nothing inside vagina.

Ectopic Pregnancy

An ectopic pregnancy occurs when a fertilized egg implants anywhere outside of the uterus (usually in the fallopian tubes). Complications include a ruptured ectopic pregnancy and hemorrhage.

1. *Causes:* The cause is not always known, but pelvic inflammatory disease with scarring and tubal ligation are contributing factors.
2. *Signs and symptoms:* severe sharp pain or cramping; absent or slight vaginal bleeding; irregular or missed period; and signs of shock.
3. *Interventions:* anticipate orders for: pregnancy test, check Hcg level, arrange for pelvic/transvaginal ultrasound, start large-bore intravenous access, set up pelvic examination, perform coagulation studies, type and screen blood, determine Rh factor, check frequent vital signs, and prepare for surgery.

Fast facts in a nutshell

Question: A 22-year-old female arrives in the emergency room complaining of right lower quadrant (RLQ) abdominal pain. What must be ruled out?
Answer: *Ectopic pregnancy, and appendicitis.*

*Notes:*____

____

____

Placenta Previa

Placenta previa occurs when the placenta implants itself in the lower uterus, thereby partially or completely covering the cervical opening.

1. *Causes:* Unknown
2. *Signs and symptoms:* painless bright red vaginal bleeding during pregnancy, and soft nontender abdomen.
3. *Interventions:* anticipate orders for: bed rest, intravenous access, monitor fetal heart tones and frequent vital signs, count menstrual pads, monitor for signs of shock, position the patient on left side, arrange for pelvic ultrasound. *PELVIC EXAM IS CONTRAINDICATED, AS IT COULD CAUSE FURTHER BLEEDING.* GET THE PATIENT TO THE BIRTH CENTER, and prepare for possible emergency C-section.

*Notes:*____

____

____

Abruptio placentae

Abruptio placentae is when the placenta breaks away from the uterine wall before delivery.

1. *Causes:* Not always known, but can be attributed to abdominal trauma or a very short umbilical cord pulling on the placenta.
2. *Signs and symptoms:* abdominal pain/cramps; profuse or concealed *dark red vaginal bleeding;* uterine contractions; fetal distress; and signs of shock.
3. *Interventions:* position patient on her left side; administer high-flow oxygen via nonrebreather mask; monitor fetal heart tones, frequent vital signs, and cardiac rhythm; anticipate orders to: begin intravenous access, perform coagulation studies, type and screen blood, and prepare for possible emergency C-section and transport to birth center.

Fast facts in a nutshell

Question: What is the major difference between placenta previa and abruptio placentae?
Answer: *Placenta previa is* painless bright red *vaginal bleeding, abruptio placentae is* painful dark red *vaginal bleeding.*

*Notes:*____

____

____

Pregnancy-Induced Hypertension (Pre-eclampsia)

Pregnancy-induced hypertension is diagnosed hypertension that occurs only during pregnancy. Once the pregnancy is over, the blood pressure is normotensive again.

1. *Causes:* Unknown.
2. *Signs and symptoms:* hypertension; headaches; edema; epigastric pain; sudden weight gain; proteinuria; double vision; uterine contractions; and vaginal bleeding.
3. *Interventions:* monitor blood pressure; perform urinalysis; arrange for transvaginal or pelvic ultrasound; bed rest; position patient on left side; monitor urine output; anticipate orders to: obtain a complete metabolic panel, a complete blood count, and a liver function test, monitor cardiac performance and fetal heart tones, begin intravenous access, prepare for possible hospital admission, take seizure precautions and consider administering intravenous magnesium sulfate.

*Notes:*____

____

____

Eclampsia

Eclampsia is a seizure associated with pre-eclampsia.

1. *Causes:* Unknown.
2. *Signs and symptoms:* seizure activity associated with pre-eclampsia symptoms, including hypertension; headaches; edema; epigastric pain; sudden weight gain; proteinuria; double vision; uterine contractions; and vaginal bleeding.
3. *Interventions:* anticipate orders to: begin intravenous access, take serum uric acid and liver function tests, perform a complete blood count and basic metabolic panel, measure hourly urine output via Foley catheter, administer anticonvulsants intravenously (e.g., magnesium sulfate), administer hydralazine intramuscularly or intravenously if diastolic blood pressure is greater than 110 mm Hg, monitor cardiac performance, level of consciousness, urinary output, and blood pressure, take seizure precautions, provide psychosocial support, and prepare for emergent delivery.

*Notes:*____

____

____

Prolapsed Cord

The cord is prolapsed when a pregnant woman comes into the emergency room in active labor and you see the cord hanging out. GET HER TO THE BIRTH CENTER IMMEDIATELY.

1. *Causes:* Unknown
2. *Signs and symptoms:* A woman in active labor with the umbilical cord presenting through the vaginal canal before the baby.
3. *Interventions:* Do **not** try to put the cord back in. Manual pressure can be applied to the baby's head by gently pushing up with the finger to relieve pressure on umbilical cord. Prepare for emergency C-section.

*Notes:*____

____

____

Trauma During Pregnancy

This trauma is the result of an injury that occurred during pregnancy.

1. *Causes:* vary individually. Shift in weight and unsteady gait do contribute to falls and injuries during pregnancy.
2. *Signs and symptoms:* vary depending on the injury. May include vaginal bleeding and ruptured membranes.
3. *Interventions:* assess uterine contractions and fetal heart tones (normal is 120–160 beat/min); place the patient in left lateral recumbent position; anticipate orders to: obtain large-bore intravenous access, administer isotonic intravenous fluids, determine presence of any amniotic fluids with pH strip, inspect vaginal opening for crowning, check for any fetal movement, palpate and determine fundal height, arrange for pelvic or transvaginal ultrasound and

CT scan, perform coagulation studies, prepare a complete blood count, type and screen blood, arrange for pelvic examination, access breath sounds for pulmonary edema, prepare for blood transfusion, and prepare for emergency C-section. NO vasopressors due to fetal compromise.

Fast facts in a nutshell

- If a pregnant patient is on backboard, tilt the client to her left side to move the uterus off the inferior vena cava (IVC).
- Consider early blood transfusion. Large quantities of isotonic fluids do not improve fetal hypoxia.
- A pregnant trauma patient can lose up to 30% of blood volume before becoming hypotensive.

*Notes:*______________________________________

____

____

Emergency Delivery

It is rare, but sometimes babies are delivered in the emergency room. Most times, we feel ill prepared. Sometimes patients don't know they are pregnant or are in denial. Just remember, women have been delivering babies naturally without hospitals and nurses since the beginning of time.

1. *Causes:* There are only three reasons to deliver a baby in the emergency room. (1) The patient in active labor did not know she was pregnant. (2) The patient is miscarrying and is less than 20 weeks pregnant. (3) The active labor patient accidentally comes to the emergency room instead of the birthing center and delivers prior to being transferred to the birthing center.
2. *Signs and symptoms:* bloody; amniotic fluid leakage; crowning or a baby's head; and an uncontrollable desire to push (patient may ask to use the bathroom).
3. *Interventions:* position the patient on her left side; administer oxygen; and visually check for crowning. If signs of imminent delivery are present, be prepared to "catch" the baby; obtain intravenous access as ordered; monitor fetal heart tones and contractions; and prepare for *rapid vaginal examination unless vaginal bleeding is present.* Vaginal bleeding due to placenta previa may cause *LIFE-THREATENING HEMORRHAGE.*
   a. *Infant resuscitation:* So you have caught the baby. Now what? Call for help if you don't have any.
      1. *Prevent heat loss by drying the baby* and wrapping him or her in warm blankets/towels; use warming light; and placing directly against mother's body and cover both.
      2. *Suctioning:* bulb suction mouth then nose. If you don't have bulb suction, use wall suction with oral Yanker adapter.
      3. *Provide oxygen.*

TABLE 13.3 The APGAR Score

Sign	0	1	2
Color	Cyanotic/blue	Body pink, blue extremities	Whole body pink
Muscle tone	Limp	Some flexion	Active movement
Respirations	Absent	Slow, irregular	Good (30–60)
Heart Rate	Absent	Slow (less than 100 bpm)	Good (100–180/hr)
Reflex Irritability (tactile stimulation)	No response	Facial grimace	Cry, cough, sneeze

4. *Stimulate:* If the drying and the suction don't work, rub the infant's back or flick/slap soles of feet. If still not breathing, use bag valve mask to assist ventilations.
5. *The APGAR Score* is used to determine fetal status. Use Table 13.3 to determine the baby's score. You want the baby to score a perfect 10.

*Notes:*______________________________

____

____

Fast facts in a nutshell

Question: Where would a 32-week-pregnant patient diagnosed with appendicitis be hurting?
Answer: *Right upper quadrant because it gets pushed up later in pregnancy.*

Question: What does gravida mean? What does para mean?
Answer: *Gravida means the number of pregnancies. Para means the number of live births.*

Fast facts in a nutshell: summary

You should now have a more defining knowledge base of obstetrical and gynecological emergencies. Be sure to locate and be familiar with all your obstetrical and gynecological equipment. Nothing is worse than running around trying to find supplies during an emergency. Be sure to practice assisting with a couple of pelvic examinations during your orientation. At first, you may feel like you need a few extra hands to assist with the examinations. Obtain a good history! This means asking questions, such as when did it start, does anything make the pain worse, how many pads did you go through today? Always be professional and respect your patient's privacy.

Chapter 14

Ocular Emergencies

INTRODUCTION

You will come across a variety of eye emergencies working in the emergency room. Some are as simple as pink eye, while others require emergency ophthalmic surgery. ***As a nurse, you must be able to differentiate between non-urgent and emergent eye complaints.*** *This chapter will guide you through the various types of eye emergencies and teach you the manifestations and interventions for each. Be sure to practice with the eye supplies available at your facility during your orientation. Familiarization with your supplies will enable you to obtain a thorough eye assessment on your patients. The providers you work with will be expecting a visual acuity on all eye complaints.* ***Document carefully and keep your eyes open;*** *you never know what you'll see next in the emergency room.*

During this part of your orientation, locate and become familiar with:

1. Wood's lamp, slit lamp, Tono-Pen or tonometer.
2. Eye exam supplies (fluorescein strips, tetracaine or proparacaine hydrochloride [Alcaine] eyedrops).
3. Visual acuity charts.
4. pH indicator strips.
5. Morgan lens and eye irrigation supplies.
6. Gentamicin ophthalmic ointment.

Fast facts in a nutshell

All patients with eye complaints need visual acuity documented.

DIAGNOSES

Central Retinal Artery Occlusion

This is a thrombus or embolus central retinal artery occlusion. There is a **one hour** window to restore blood flow. **This is A TRUE OCULAR EMERGENCY!**

1. *Causes:* Just as with a stroke, thrombi or emboli can occlude the retinal artery, cutting off the blood supply to the eye.
2. *Signs and symptoms:* sudden/painless/unilateral/complete loss of vision; dilated nonreactive pupil; and pale fundus.

3. *Interventions:* check the patient's visual acuity; obtain eye exam equipment; anticipate orders to: obtain intravenous access, administer vasodilators (e.g., intravenous nitroglycerin) and anticoagulants, arrange ophthalmology consult, and prepare for surgery.

*Notes:*____

____

____

Glaucoma

Acute open-angle glaucoma occurs from optic nerve damage.

1. *Causes:* It starts with blockage of the outflow of fluid from the anterior chamber. This results in elevated intraocular pressure leading to optic nerve damage.
2. *Signs and symptoms:* diminished vision; deep eye pain; nausea and vomiting; tearing; photophobia; cloudy cornea; semidilated nonreactive pupils; red conjunctiva; and increased ocular pressure.
3. *Interventions:* obtain visual acuity; anticipate provider will monitor ocular pressure; administer myotic eyedrops/topical beta antagonists as ordered, and obtain ophthalmologist consult.

*Notes:*____

____

____

Corneal Abrasions

These are scratches/abrasions to the clear surface (cornea) of the eye with or without foreign bodies.

1. *Causes:* Practically anything that can scratch the skin can scratch the cornea. In most cases, it is some type of foreign body.
2. *Signs and symptoms:* eye pain; corneal irregularity; no corneal luster; photophobia; copious tearing; and foreign body sensation.
3. *Interventions:* assess visual acuity; obtain eye exam equipment (eye kit, Wood's lamp); anticipate orders to: administer antibiotic eyedrops or ointment, update tetanus/ diphtheria shot, administer oral analgesics, and provide ophthalmologist referral.

*Notes:*____

____

____

Detached Retina

The retina is made of two layers (outer pigmented and inner sensory). A detached retina occurs when these layers separate.

1. *Causes:* vitreous humor leakage; eye trauma; inflammatory disorders; and uncontrolled diabetes.
2. *Signs and symptoms:* painless decreased vision; smoky or cloudy vision; flashing lights; and peripheral floaters (black dots)/"curtain effect."

3. *Interventions:* check visual acuity; position patient supinely; anticipate orders to: arrange ophthalmology consult, administer mydriatic drops to dilate pupil, apply bilateral eye patches, and prepare for surgery and admission.

*Notes:*____

____

____

Conjunctivitis/Pink Eye

This is an inflammation of the conjunctiva. Bacterial and viral conjunctivitis are highly contagious.

1. *Causes:* bacteria, viruses, chemicals, or allergies.
2. *Signs and symptoms:* itchy eyes; photophobia; normal visual acuity; purulent or serous eye discharge; reddened conjunctiva; and copious tearing.
3. *Interventions:* assess visual acuity; anticipate orders to: instill topical anesthetic, obtain fluorescein staining supplies and Wood's lamp, and instill ophthalmic antibiotic eyedrops or ointment.

Fast facts in a nutshell

Because conjunctivitis is so contagious, discharge instructions should include: strict hand washing after touching eye area, no sharing of hand towels, discarding current eye make-up, and disinfecting sunglasses.

*Notes:*____

Penetrating Trauma

Penetrating trauma requires immediate ophthalmology consult. Protruding objects are NOT to be removed, but carefully secured in place.

1. *Causes:* Vary. You name it, but anything from knives and bullets to nails shot through nail guns. Practically anything with enough force behind it can cause penetrating trauma to the eye.
2. *Signs and symptoms:* irregular pupil shape; impaired visual acuity; and decreased intraocular pressure.
3. *Interventions:* cover injured eye with metal or plastic patch and patch other eye to reduce eye movement; put patient in semi-Fowler's position; anticipate orders to administer pain medication and give tetanus/diphtheria injection.

*Notes:*____

Blunt Trauma Blow-Out Fractures

This is a fracture of the orbital floor.

1. *Causes:* inferior orbital rim trauma.
2. *Signs and symptoms:* change in gaze; diplopia; ecchymosis; subconjunctival hemorrhage; paresthesia; periorbital edema; crepitus; and inability to look up due to inferior rectus/inferior oblique muscle entrapment.
3. *Interventions:* apply ice pack; anticipate orders to: administer pain medications, arrange for orbital X-rays or CT scan, put patient in semi-Fowler's position, and prepare for possible admission or surgery.

*Notes:*____

____

____

Hyphema

Hyphema is a hemorrhage into the anterior chamber of eye that results in corneal blood staining, secondary glaucoma, visual impairment, or loss of an eye.

1. *Causes:* eye trauma.
2. *Signs and symptoms:* blood in anterior chamber of eye; impaired visual acuity; and "seeing red" or floater.
3. *Interventions:* elevate the patient's head of the bed to 60 degrees; gently patch both eyes; anticipate orders to arrange immediate ophthalmology consult, monitor intraocular pressure, and administer mannitol or osmotic diuretic for increased intraocular pressure.

Notes: ____

____

____

Chemical Burns

Chemical burns are the result of contact with ACID or ALKALI solutions. Alkali is more serious and can result in loss of vision. **THIS IS A TRUE EYE EMERGENCY!**

1. *Causes:* foreign chemical contact with the eye.
2. *Signs and symptom:* eye pain; visual disturbances; corneal whitening; copious tearing; surrounding skin irritation; and corneal ulceration.
3. *Interventions:* assess visual acuity; check pH with litmus paper; immediately apply copious amounts of normal saline/lactated Ringer's; anticipate orders to: maintain continuous irrigation until pH of the eye is 6.9 to 7.2, administer ophthalmic ointment, and arrange ophthalmology referral.

Fast facts in a nutshell

Acid burns usually require 30- to 60-minute irrigations. Alkali burns may take 1 hour or longer to irrigate. This procedure gets fluid everywhere. You will need to give the patient a gown, place them in the modified Trendelenburg position, and place a couple of Chux under their head that drain into a basin on the floor.

Notes: ____

____

____

Fast facts in a nutshell: summary

Eye emergencies occur pretty routinely in the emergency room. It is vital to recognize which ones are emergent and which ones are nonurgent. Be sure to document pupil size, pupil reaction to light, pupil symmetry, and visual acuity. You should now be more confident in recognizing the symptoms and treatments for the various types of eye emergencies and in treating them. However, you need to practice with the current eye supplies at your facility to truly complete your ocular emergency orientation.

Chapter 15

Orthopedic and Wound Care Emergencies

INTRODUCTION

You will definitely see all kinds of orthopedic and wound emergencies in the emergency room. You need to be familiar with many difference pieces of orthopedic equipment. In addition to using the equipment, the emergency room nurse is also responsible for teaching the patient how to use the orthopedic equipment. For cast of Ortho-Glass type splinting, I recommend training from the manufacturer's representative. ***Most manufacturers will send someone to your facility to demonstrate their products and allow employees to practice applying the splints.*** *Most emergency room technicians are qualified to apply splints for you, but the nurse must ensure the work was done properly. This chapter will provide a brief overview of the different orthopedic and wound care emergency situations you may come across in the emergency room, and how to handle them.*

During this part of your orientation, locate and become familiar with:

1. Ace wraps, splinting, and casting materials.
2. Crutches.
3. Hare traction splints, and Buck's traction.
4. Tube gauze.
5. Finger traps and weights.
6. Suture supplies and dressing supplies.
7. Medications to know: lidocaine 1 or 2% (with or without epinephrine), morphine, meperidine (Demerol), hydrocodone (Lortab), oxycodone (Percocet), and acetaminophen (Tylenol) with codeine.

DIAGNOSES

Strains

A strain is a pull or tear to a tendon or muscle.

1. *Causes:* injury resulting in a pull or tear to a tendon.
2. *Signs and symptoms:* pain; swelling; ecchymosis; edema; point tenderness; spasm; and decreased range of motion.
3. *Interventions:* (PRICE) Protect (splint, cast, sling), Rest, Ice, Compression (ace wrap), Elevate; X-ray; instruct patient on use of crutches for light to no weight bearing; and arrange orthopedic follow-up.

Notes: ______________________________________

____

____

Sprains

A sprain is a pull or tear to a ligament, commonly in the knees, ankles, and shoulders.

1. *Causes:* injury resulting in a pull or tear to a ligament.
2. *Signs and symptoms:* pain; swelling; ecchymosis; edema; point tenderness; spasm; and decreased range of motion.
3. *Interventions:* (PRICE) Protect (splint, cast, sling), Rest, Ice, Compression (ace wrap), Elevate; X-ray; instruct patient on light to no weight bearing (crutches); and arrange orthopedic follow-up.

*Notes:*____

____

____

Fractures

A fracture is a broken bone.

1. *Types*
   a. Closed: skin intact.
   b. Open: broken bone with break in the skin surrounding the fracture. Patient is at high risk for developing an infection in the bone (osteomyelitis).
   c. Avulsion: Insertion site bone fragment breaks away due to forceful muscle contraction.
   d. Comminuted: two or more bone fragments.

   e. Depressed: flat bone injury due to blunt trauma.
   f. Greenstick: incomplete compression force-type fracture (common in school-age children).
   g. Spiral: twisting injury.
   h. Oblique: linear oblique fracture.
   i. Transverse: horizontal linear fracture.
   j. Segmented: broken in two or more places.
   k. Salter-Harris: fracture involving the growth plate.
   l. Boxer fracture: occurs to the 4th or 5th metacarpals after punching type injury.
2. *Causes:* injury resulting in a break to the bone.
3. *Signs and symptoms:* pain; tenderness; swelling; redness; ecchymosis; deformity; shortening/rotation in hip fracture; decreased range of motion; muscle spasm; weak or absent pulses; pallor; and shock.
4. *Interventions:* immobilize; assist in applying traction for femur fracture; cover open fractures with sterile saline soaked dressing; (PRICE) Protect (splint, cast, sling) Rest, Ice, Compression (ace wrap), Elevate; X-ray; no weight bearing (crutches); prepare for possible closed reduction; give nothing by mouth; give instructions for possible surgical repair; teach cast care instructions and crutch training; check peripheral pulses; anticipate orders to start intravenous access; possibly give intravenous fluids and tetanus immunization if open fracture; administer pain medication and evaluate effectiveness; and arrange orthopedic follow-up.

Fast facts in a nutshell

Question: How long does it take a bone to heal?
Answer: *About 6 weeks.*

Question: What other X-ray should be ordered for the patient who has bilateral heel fractures after falling 13′ off a ladder and landing on his feet?
Answer: *Check the L-spine.*

Question: Which bones, if broken, can lead to hemorrhagic shock?
Answer: *Pelvis and femur.*

Question: How much blood can be lost in one femur fracture?
Answer: *Up to 1500 ml.*

Question: When applying a thumb spica Ortho-Glass splint, how should you position the hand?
Answer: *As if the patient were holding a cup or soda can.*

Notes: ______________________________

____

____

Dislocations and Subluxations

Dislocations and subluxations occur when a joint is pulled out of place.

1. *Causes:* injury or movement resulting in joint dislocation.
2. *Signs and symptoms:* severe joint pain; joint deformity/asymmetry; decreased or absent range of motion; weak or absent pulse; edema; and shortening of extremity.
3. *Interventions:* anticipate orders to: obtain X-ray films, prepare for conscious sedation for closed reduction, apply ice pack, start intravenous access, prepare a neurovascular assessment, immobilize joint post reduction, and obtain post reduction X-ray.

Notes: ____

____

____

Amputation

Amputation is a partial or complete separation of a limb.

1. *Causes:* injury/trauma resulting in separation of a limb.
2. *Signs and symptoms:* completely or partially detached extremity.
3. *Interventions:* wrap amputated part in sterile saline-soaked gauze and place in sterile plastic bag. NEVER put amputated part directly on ice. Control bleeding; apply sterile

saline-soaked sterile dressing to amputation site; anticipate orders to: administer pain meds/antibiotics/tetanus immunization and evaluate effectiveness of medications, and prepare for surgery.

*Notes:*____

____

____

Compartment Syndrome

This occurs when a compartment of the limb becomes full of fluid or blood, thereby hindering circulation to that extremity.

1. *Causes:* usually occurs with trauma.
2. *Signs and symptoms:* the 5 P's: Pain, Paresthesia, Pulseless, Paralysis, and Pallor.
3. *Treatments:* administer anti-inflammatory drugs as ordered; elevate the affected limb; and prepare for emergency fasciotomy.

*Notes:*____

____

____

Lacerations

Lacerations are cuts or breaks in the skin.

1. *Causes:* Everything from pieces of glass, knives, and razors to umbrellas, coffee tables, and baseball bats. You name it; almost anything can cause a laceration.
2. *Signs and symptoms:* bleeding, cut, and open wound. An arterial laceration will intermittently squirt blood with each pulse. If a vein is cut, it will constantly ooze. Superficial lacerations are easily repaired in the emergency room. Deep wounds through the muscle fascia or tendons may require a plastic surgeon.
3. *Interventions:* apply pressure to control bleeding; update tetanus shot if greater than five years since last one. Cleanse wound with ChloraPrep or Sure-Cleanse. Prepare patient for wound closure with Dermabond, Steri-strips, or sutures per provider order. Bandage accordingly.

Fast facts in a nutshell

Question: When setting up for suture repair of the ear, nose, penis, fingers or toes, should you use lidocaine with epinephrine?
Answer: *No.*

Question: What supplies are needed for suture set-up?
Answer: *Suture tray, sutures, betadine/ChloraPrep, saline, lidocaine, Chux, and sterile gloves.*

Question: What are two shots that can be given in the deltoid?
Answer: *Tetanus/diphtheria and the flu shot.*

Question: A 36-year-old female comes in complaining of being bitten by a mouse. Should you give rabies vaccine?
Answer: *No, rodents don't carry rabies.*

Question: If actually contracted, is rabies fatal without proper vaccination?
Answer: *Yes.*

*Notes:*______________________________

____

____

Burns

A burn is a breakdown in the skin.

1. *Causes:* chemicals; sun; heat; radiation; fire; or even cold substances like dry ice.
2. *Signs and symptoms:*
   a. 1st degree: superficial pink or redness; pain; and warmth to area.
   b. 2nd degree: redness; blistering; break in 1st layer of skin down to second layer of skin; and pain.
   c. 3rd degree: white areas or charred black areas to skin; painless; all layers of skin affected; and possibly fat, muscle and bone involvement.
3. *Interventions:* check ABCs first. Patient may have smoke/burn inhalation or carbon monoxide poisoning. Cover burns

with sterile nonadherent dressings; give pain medication as ordered; cleanse burns with ChloraPrep and saline; and apply silver sulfadiazine (Silvadene) cream, nonadherent, or wet to dry dressings. If a major burn, prepare for admission to burn center.

Figure 15.1 shows the rules of nines for burn victims. This is a fast way to determine a patient's percentage of burned surfaces.

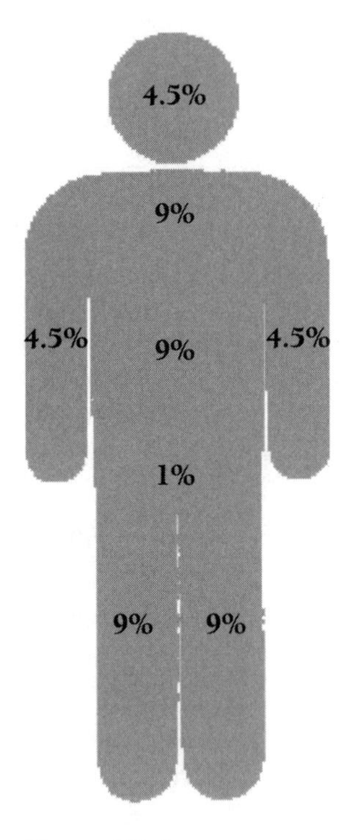

Figure 15.1

*Notes:*____

____

____

Fast facts in a nutshell: summary

You now have a better understanding of orthopedic and wound care emergencies, their symptoms, and treatments. Be sure to familiarize yourself with the orthopedic and wound care supplies at your local facility. Thoroughly document your assessments, being sure to include distal pulses, capillary refills, deformities, symmetry, if bleeding is controlled, and when and how the injury occurred. Use personal protective equipment, especially with arterial bleeds. Arterial bleeds have been known to squirt across the room. In case this happens and your clothes get soiled, it is also a good idea to keep an extra pair of scrubs in your locker.

Chapter 16

Pediatric Emergencies

INTRODUCTION

Children can be some of the most delightful and yet scariest patients you'll ever meet. Why scary? For 2 reasons. First, ***children can't always tell you what is wrong.*** *So you must assess them well and listen to parents; they generally know when something is wrong with their babies. Second,* ***children may look okay when they are actually in distress*** *because they are good at compensating. When they can no longer compensate, they deteriorate rapidly. This is called the plateau effect. This doesn't leave the emergency room staff with much time to resuscitate them. Therefore, you must treat them aggressively at the early signs of distress, which include tachycardia and increased respirations. Hypotension is a late sign, which is followed by rapid deterioration. You will learn about this extensively during your pediatric advanced life support (PALS) course.* ***Pediatric emergency nursing really is a specialty of its own,*** *but this chapter will provide you with some of the basic pediatric emergency nursing tools you will need.*

During this part of your orientation, locate and become familiar with:

1. Braslow tape and cart/bag.
2. Where to take a pediatric advanced life support class.
3. Kilogram/pound conversion.
4. Pediatric Tylenol and Motrin doses.
5. Pediatric vital signs.
6. Papoose board.
7. Intra-osseous needle, also known as I.O. needle, output placement and use.
8. Review hospital policy for consent to treat minors.
9. Stickers, popsicles, coloring crayons, and toys, as these are great for passing time and bribing.

Fast facts in a nutshell

When children deteriorate, they generally deteriorate more rapidly than adults.

Table 16.1 lists all of the pediatric vital signs according to age group. You will need to know these by heart, so it is a good idea to familiarize yourself with these vital signs during your orientation. Basically, the younger the child, the lower the blood pressure and higher the heart and respirations will be.

TABLE 16.1 Pediatric Vital Signs

Age	Systolic Blood Pressure	Heart Rate	Respirations
Infant (0–1 year)	70–92	85–205	30–60
Toddler (1–3 years)	72–96	100–190	24–40
Preschooler (3–5 years)	76–100	60–140	22–34
School age (5–10 years)	80–110	60–140	18–30
Adolescent (older than 10 years)	90–120	60–100	12–20

Fast facts in a nutshell

Obtain blood pressure on children 4 years of age and older. Don't use the word "blood" pressure, as it scares them. Tell them you're going to give their arm a hug with an arm-hugging machine or check their arm muscles.

Fever

In children, a fever is defined as a rectal temp of 100.4° or higher. Infants younger than 3 months of age with fever are at high risk for having a serious bacterial infection, such as sepsis or meningitis. A febrile child without an obvious source of fever requires an extensive evaluation and possible admission.

1. *Causes:* otitis media; pneumonia; viral infections; gastroenteritis; bacteremia; meningitis; and upper respiratory infections.
2. *Signs and symptoms:* poor feeding; rectal temperature greater than 100.4°; irritability; lethargy; dry mucous membranes; decreased tear production; sunken or bulging fontanel; tachycardia; and tachypnea.
3. *Interventions:* anticipate orders to: give antipyretic medications (acetaminophen [Tylenol] = 15 mg/kg, ibuprofen [Motrin] = 10 mg/kg) by mouth or suppository, administer intravenous fluids for dehydration, and monitor temperature.

Fast facts in a nutshell

- Sepsis work-up in infants younger than 3 months of age includes labs, chest X-ray; and lumbar puncture. Remember when positioning patient for a lumbar puncture, there should be no chin to chest, as this might occlude the airway. Instead, curve shoulders (not the head) forward.
- Fluids after a lumbar puncture may prevent headache in a young child.
- Children's ibuprofen (Motrin) is not given to children younger than 6 months of age.
- A 4-year-old with gastroenteritis who is discharged from the emergency department should be encouraged to drink small sips of clear liquids as much as he can tolerate to make up fluid loss. Popsicles and Jell-O are kid-friendly choices.

*Notes:*______________________________________

____

____

Epiglottitis

Epiglottitis is a rapid swelling and inflammation of the epiglottis that can lead to a life-threatening airway obstruction. It commonly occurs in children 2 to 6 years of age.

1. *Causes:* acute bacterial infection of the epiglottis.
2. *Signs and symptoms:* sudden onset (2–4 hours); drooling; dysphagia or refusing to drink; inspiratory stridor (abnormal sound over trachea); respiratory distress; tripod position; muffled voice; hoarseness; high fever; sore throat; and anxiety.
3. *Interventions:* decrease stimulation (don't make them cry); maintain position of comfort; permit caregiver to stay with child; give oxygen by any method tolerated (blow-by); anticipate orders to: prepare for intubation, start intravenous access after securing airway and administer antibiotics.

*Notes:*______________________________________

____

____

Bronchiolitis

Bronchiolitis is a viral infection of the bronchioles, with increased mucous secretion that results in mucus plugging and air trapping.

1. *Causes:* the respiratory syncytial virus (RSV). It affects mostly infants younger than one year of age.
2. *Signs and symptoms:* cough; runny nose; poor feeding; respiratory distress; pallor; retractions; grunting; nasal flaring; wheezing; apnea spells; and fever.
3. *Interventions:* anticipate orders to: arrange for chest X-ray, administer fluids by mouth or intravenously, isolate, give oxygen, use nebulizers, administer racemic epinephrine, ribavirin, place head of bed up, and prepare for admission, if severe.

*Notes:*____

____

____

Croup

Croup is inflammation and edema of the vocal cords, trachea, and bronchi. It most commonly affects children from 6 months to 3 years of age at night in late fall to early winter.

1. *Causes:* a viral illness.
2. *Signs and symptoms:* barking cough (like a barking seal); inspiratory stridor; hoarse voice; respiratory distress; low fever; and tachycardia.

3. *Interventions:* anticipate orders to: administer cool mist oxygen, give fluids by mouth or intravenously, and give steroids and racemic epinephrine.

*Notes:*____

____

____

Shunted Hydrocephalus

Hydrocephalus is commonly caused by obstructed cerebrospinal fluid, which leads to a dilated ventricular system. A shunt is inserted to drain the fluid away from the cranium to the peritoneum or the left atria. Ventriculoperitoneal shunts are the most common. A child might present to the emergency department as a result of infection or malfunction of the shunt.

1. *Causes:* obstruction to flow of cerebrospinal fluid.
2. *Signs and symptoms:* fever; behavioral changes; erythema or fluid along shunt tubing track; meningeal signs; acute abdominal pain; diarrhea; peritonitis; increased intracranial pressure; seizure activity; and headache.
3. *Interventions:* maintain support of airway/breathing/circulation (ABCs); elevate head of bed up 30°; anticipate orders to: administer intravenous fluids (often fluid is restricted), diuretics, analgesics, anticonvulsants, and antibiotics and monitor their effectiveness, anticipate need of removal of cerebrospinal fluid from shunt, take seizure precautions, and monitor cardiac performance, respiratory rate, and continuous pulse oximetry.

Notes: ______________________________

____

____

Child Abuse

Remember that child abuse includes physical, emotional, psychological, and sexual abuse, as well as neglect.

1. *Causes:* many nurses find it impossible to understand what causes a person to harm a child, but it can happen in any socioeconomic class and is usually brought on by the adult's inability to cope with stress.
2. *Signs and symptoms:* bruise or fractures in various stages of healing; burn patterns from cigarettes or hot water; human bite marks; head injuries from direct blows or vigorous shaking, alopecia, lip bruising or laceration; loss of teeth; hyphema; corneal abrasion; retinal hemorrhage; orbital fracture; periorbital hematoma; spiral fractures from twisting injuries; and abdominal trauma (abdominal distention, nausea and vomiting, and abdominal pain).
   a. A history may provide vital clues. Always interview parents individually, and, if possible, the child separately.
      1. Is there any preexisting medical condition that explains present injuries?
      2. Does caregiver's history match the mechanism of injury?
      3. Does caregiver deny knowledge of injury occurrence?
      4. Any inconsistent history changes?

5. Any delay in seeking medical attention?
6. Any history of unexplained suspicious injuries?
7. Has the caregiver bypassed closer medical facilities to reach yours?
8. Is anyone else besides the parents caring for the child?

3. *Signs and symptoms of neglect:* malnourishment; poor hygiene; inappropriate dress; inadequate medical care; bald patches on infant head from being left in crib in one position for long time; abandonment; numerous dental problems; lack of supervision; and educational neglect.
4. *Signs and symptoms of sexual abuse:* genital/rectal trauma; vaginal/rectal bleeding or pain; vaginal discharge; unusual vaginal/rectal dilation; increased rectal pigmentation; dysuria; frequent urination; foreign bodies in vagina/urethra/rectum; pregnancy; difficulty ambulating; sexually transmitted diseases; and bowel incontinence.
5. *Interventions:* anticipate orders to: perform labs (HIV, rapid plasma reagin, amylase, lipase), arrange for CT scan, ultrasound, and X-rays (complete skeletal survey in child younger than two years of age), provide safe environment, treat injuries, provide emotional support to caregiver and child, remain nonjudgmental, explain tests and procedures, allow caregiver to remain with child except during interview, refer to social services, report all suspected cases to child protective services, complete appropriate paperwork, carefully document shape, size, location, and appearance of all injuries, and document reports from caregiver and child word for word in quotation marks. For suspected sexual abuse, lab protocol may include collecting vaginal/cervical/rectal culture; vaginal/rectal fluids; pregnancy test; ABO-antigen typing; and hair specimen.

Fast facts in a nutshell

- Parents from any socioeconomic class may be child abusers.
- The abused child does not cry when parent leaves the room.

Question: Which is not considered child abuse?

a. Burns from the ankles down
b. Missing hair on head
c. Belt marks
d. Bruises on bilateral elbows and knees

Answer: *d is correct.*

Notes: ___

Congenital Heart Diseases

There are several different types; they are classified as left-to-right shunts (acyanotic) or right-to-left shunts (cyanotic).

- Left-to-right shunts (acyanotic): atrial septal defect, atrioventricular septal defect, ventricular septal defect, and patent ductus arteriosus.
- Right-to-left shunts (cyanotic): tetralogy of Fallot, tricuspid atresia, transposition of the great vessels, aortic stenosis, pulmonic stenosis, and coarctation of the aorta.

1. *Causes:* Unknown.
2. *Signs and symptoms:* cyanosis with feeding or activity; decreased urine; edema; cardiomegaly; hepatomegaly; developmental delays; murmurs; tachycardia; bradycardia; tachypnea; dyspnea; cough; respiratory distress; clubbing of fingers or toes; poor peripheral circulation; mottling of extremities; syncope; and "tet spells" (squatting position to relieve dyspnea).
3. *Interventions:* remember the ABCs; provide basic life support if indicated; anticipate orders for: arterial blood gas levels, electrocardiogram and echocardiogram, possible cardiac catheter procedure, allow child to be in position of comfort, administer oxygen, use bag valve mask (BVM) if needed, start intravenous access, set head of bed at 30°, administer medications (digitalis, diuretics, analgesics, and sedatives) as ordered, limit noxious stimuli, and keep comfortably warm.

*Notes:*____

____

____

Nursemaid's Elbow (Radial Head Subluxation)

Nursemaid's elbow is a subluxation of the elbow.

1. *Causes:* commonly occurs when a child younger than 5 years of age is grabbed by the forearm to pull up or swing.
2. *Signs and symptoms:* no use of suspected arm after pulling mechanism of the forearm. Child may guard arm. No signs of trauma noted.

3. *Intervention:* assist with simple reduction; arrange for X-ray; administer analgesics as ordered; and apply ice pack.

*Notes:*____

____

____

Sudden Infant Death Syndrome

This is the most common cause of death in infants between 1 month and 1 year old.

1. *Causes:* Unknown. Studies show that placing an infant on his or her back to sleep helps reduce the risk of sudden infant death syndrome.
2. *Signs and symptoms:* most caregivers report finding an infant in a crib not breathing or face down in crib. Autopsy fails to reveal cause of death.
3. *Interventions:* attempt to resuscitate using pediatric advance life support protocol, unless obvious rigor mortis has set in. **Refer parents to SIDS support group.**

*Notes:*____

____

____

Intussusception

Intussusception occurs when a segment of the intestines folds over on itself like a telescope. It most commonly occurs in children younger than 1 year of age. Intussusception can lead to obstruction, edema, and bowel necrosis.

1. *Causes:* Unknown, although existing medical conditions may be factors.
2. *Signs and symptoms:* change in eating or bowel pattern; colic; crying; drawing up knees; vomiting; currant-jelly-like red stool; recent infection; and palpable sausage-like mass.
3. *Interventions:* anticipate orders to: use nasogastric tube for decompression, administer intravenous fluids, give antibiotics, and prepare for surgical reduction, if needed.

*Notes:*____

____

____

Fast fact in a nutshell

- After visiting her grandfather who has shingles, a little girl develops a rash. The rash is most likely chickenpox.

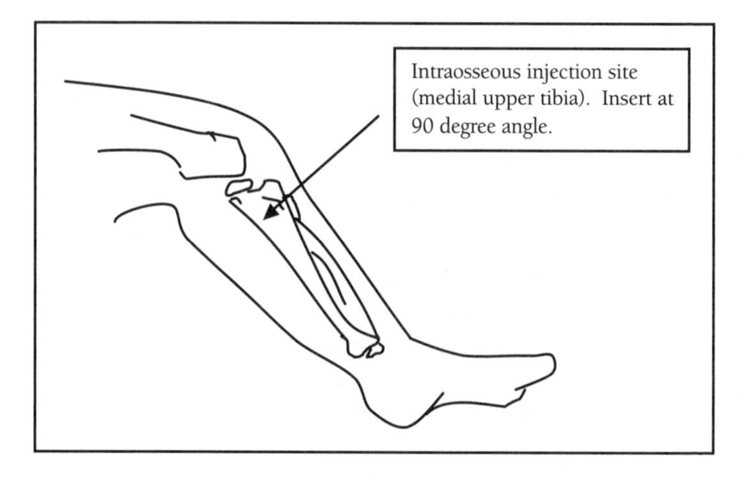

Figure 16.1

Figure 16.1 is a picture of an intraosseous injection site. This site is primarily used if intravenous access is unobtainable after two attempts during an emergency situation.

Fast facts in a nutshell: summary

Pediatric emergency nursing is its own specialty. For the general emergency nurse, the basic information in this chapter will see you through most problems. Be sure to always take account of differences between children and adults. Pediatric patients have different vital signs, deteriorate more rapidly than adults, become dehydrated more easily, and can run higher fevers. All pediatric patient medication doses are based on weight in kilograms. Remember that children can not always tell you what is wrong. Therefore, it is up to the nurse to obtain an accurate history and detailed physical assessment. If you're ever unsure of something, ask a coworker and go find the answer. The pediatric patient is not just a patient; he or she is someone's child! Sometimes, the toughest challenge is defusing the hysterical parent's anger or anxiety. Parents don't always realize they are hindering or delaying care when they panic. If the situation cannot be defused, don't waste time. Have another coworker or manager handle the parent, leaving you to care for the child. You now have the knowledge base to diagnose and handle pediatric emergencies. Be careful, these little patients know how to pull on your heart strings.

Chapter 17

Respiratory Emergencies

INTRODUCTION

Of all emergencies, respiratory problems must be treated first. Without a patent airway and breathing, your patient will die—and nothing else matters. Therefore, as an emergency nurse, you must be able to recognize and rapidly respond to any respiratory emergency. This chapter will take you through the most common respiratory conditions seen in the emergency room. After reviewing it, you will be able to recognize the various types of respiratory emergencies and know how to intervene.

During this part of your orientation, locate and become familiar with:

1. Ambu-bags, nasal cannulas, nonrebreather masks, and nebulizers.
2. Intubation equipment.
3. Chest tubes and drainage systems.
4. Ventilators, BiPAP, C-PAP.

5. Reading ABGs.
6. Drugs to know: methylprednisolone sodium succinate (Solu-Medrol), dexamethasone (Decadron), levofloxacin (Levaquin), magnesium sulfate, albuterol, ipratropium bromide (Atrovent), and levobuterol hydrochloride (Xopenex).

Fast facts in a nutshell

Always treat airway first, breathing next, and then circulation. Just remember ABC.

DIAGNOSES

Airway Obstruction

These can be divided into partial, complete, and upper or lower airway obstructions.

1. *Causes:* Vary depending on circumstance. Anything from food to coins to a swollen tongue can occlude an airway.
2. *Signs and symptoms:* respiratory distress; dyspnea; choking sensation; drooling; wheezing; decreased or no air movement; aphasia; tachycardia; tachypnea; cough; chest retractions; pallor or cyanosis; and cardiopulmonary arrest.
3. *Interventions:* clear airway; initiate basic life-support techniques for foreign-object obstruction; anticipate foreign body removal with Magill forceps by provider and orders to: administer oxygen, measure pulse oximetry, if alert and

coughing place in high-Fowler's position; prepare for intubation and possible cricothyrotomy or tracheostomy; monitor airway patency changes; and monitor respirations.

> **Fast facts in a nutshell**
>
> **Question:** A child swallowed a quarter, is drooling, and has an unusual cough. What is your concern?
> **Answer:** *Airway obstruction (remember your ABCs)*

*Notes:*____

____

____

Chronic Obstructive Pulmonary Disease

COPD is an irreversible chronic obstructive airway disease. A patient with COPD will have elevated carbon dioxide levels. Over time, the elevated carbon dioxide levels will make the patient dependent on lower PAO_2 level changes (hypoxia) to regulate ventilations. Therefore, if you deliver high-flow oxygen, the patient will lose his or her hypoxic respiratory drive **and stop breathing!**

1. *Causes:* enlargement of the alveoli; loss of lung tissue elasticity; and destruction of alveolar wall. This chronic lung

damage is associated with emphysema, chronic bronchitis, and cigarette smoking.

2. *Signs and symptoms:* dyspnea; tachypnea; pursed-lip breathing; wheezing; crackles; tripod position; use of accessory muscles; barrel chest; tachycardia; hypertension; confusion; cyanosis; premature ventricular contractions; and acute respiratory failure.
3. *Interventions:* anticipate orders to: obtain and monitor arterial blood gases, administer 1 to 2 liters of low-flow oxygen because of carbon dioxide retention, position head of bed up 90%, apply bilevel positive airway pressure (BiPAP), give nebulizer treatments and corticosteroids, give high-flow oxygen via nonrebreather only if patient is in severe respiratory distress.

*Notes:*____

____

____

Asthma

Asthma is a reversible chronic reactive airway disease. It is a complex inflammatory process characterized by airway inflammation and structural changes. Asthma is classified into four categories. Decrease in pulse oxygen is a late sign.

1. *Causes:* A hypersensitive immune system that causes the airways to inflame and swell when exposed to certain triggers. The triggers vary from person to person, but common triggers include dust; pollen; pet dander; exercise; cigarette

smoke; upper respiratory infections; and gastroesophageal reflux disease.

2. *Signs and symptoms:* vary by category.
   a. *Mild intermittent:* expiratory wheezing; pulse oximeter reading of 95 to 100; and cough.
   b. *Mild persistent:* inspiratory and expiratory wheezing; pulse oxygen of 95 to 100; and cough.
   c. *Moderate persistent:* inspiratory wheezing; expirations diminished; cough; use of accessory muscles; retractions; nasal flaring; and tripod position.
   d. *Severe persistent:* expirations diminished; no breath sounds; diaphoresis; dusky pallor or cyanotic skin color; pulse oxygen reading of less than 95; bradypnea or periods of apnea; and drowsiness or altered mental status.
3. *Interventions:* anticipate orders to: give oxygen, nebulizer treatment, steroids, and magnesium sulfate, hydrate the patient, apply bilevel positive airway pressure, and intubate in late stage.

Fast facts in a nutshell

- In the reversal of bronchospasms, the breath sounds go from diminished to louder to clear.
- Don't give diphenhydramine hydrochloide (Benadryl), propranolol (Inderal), or morphine sulfate to asthmatics.
- The optimal peak expiratory flow rate is greater than 80% of predicted or personal best.

*Notes:*____

____

____

Pulmonary Embolus (PE)

Pulmonary embolus is a complete or partial thrombus blockage of the pulmonary artery that results in systemic hypoxia.

1. *Causes:* blood clots or emboli.
2. *Signs and symptoms:* sudden dyspnea and tachypnea; respiratory distress; anxiety; restlessness; confusion; chest pain; cough; hemoptysis; wheezing; diaphoresis; pallor from the nipple line up; fever; hypotension; right-sided congestive heart failure with peaked p-waves on electrocardiogram; jugular vein distention (JVD); cyanosis; and respiratory arrest.
3. *Interventions:* anticipate orders to: give oxygen, obtain pulmonary angiography or pulmonary ventilation/perfusion scan, apply bilevel positive airway pressure, use bag valve mask for ventilatory assistance, prepare for intubation, start intravenous access, administer intravenous fluids and anticoagulants, use intravenous or inhaled bronchodilators, and give analgesics, antidysrhythmics, and thrombolytic and platelet aggregation inhibitor therapy.

Fast facts in a nutshell

Question: When a 27-year-old female arrives in the emergency department complaining of sudden onset of shortness of breath, what question should you ask?
Answer: *Is she currently taking any birth control medication?*

Notes: ____

____

____

Spontaneous Pneumothorax

Spontaneous pneumothorax is an air leak in the pleural space that results in partial or total collapse of the lung.

1. *Causes:* not always known. However, chronic obstructive pulmonary disease, asthma, cystic fibrosis, tuberculosis, pneumonia, lung cancer, interstitial lung disease, inhaled substance abuse, barometric pressure changes (scuba divers, pilots), toxic drug pentamidine, smoking, and immunodeficiency disease all attribute to spontaneous pneumothoraxes.
2. *Signs and symptoms:* dyspnea; tachypnea; tachycardia; sudden pleuritic chest pain; anxiety; restlessness; diminished or absent breath sounds on affected side; pallor; hypotension

if severe; subcutaneous emphysema; palpitations; or asymptomatic (if small).
3. *Interventions:* place in high-Fowler's position; prepare for needle thoracostomy or chest tube insertion; and administer pain meds as ordered.

Fast facts in a nutshell

If a tall, thin young adult states, "I suddenly coughed and became short of breath," think spontaneous pneumothorax.

Pneumonia

Pneumonia is an acute inflammatory reaction that results in fluid and cellular debris accumulating in segments and lobes of the lung.

1. *Causes:* aspiration, bacterial, or viral infections.
2. *Signs and symptoms:* productive cough; fever (acute onset); chills; pleuritic chest pain; dyspnea; tachypnea; respiratory distress; tachycardia; confusion; altered level of consciousness; crackles; wheezing; diminished breath sounds; and weight loss.
3. *Interventions:* anticipate orders to: obtain intravenous access, take blood cultures, administer antibiotics, rehydrate,

use nebulizers, order complete blood count and chest X-ray, and give antipyretics (if fever).

Fast facts in a nutshell

Question: What is the major pulmonary cause of septic shock?
Answer: *Acute bacterial pneumonia.*

*Notes:*____

____

____

Burn Inhalation

If a patient has burns to the face, consider the possibility of burns to the large and small airways. Patients may appear stable initially, but remember that burns swell quickly, resulting in rapid loss of airway.

1. *Causes:* burns to face, neck, chest, mouth, or airway.
2. *Signs and symptoms:* black-tinged sputum; dry mucous membranes; rales; rhonchi; and dry nonproductive cough.
3. *Interventions:* prepare for emergent intubation; apply non-rebreather oxygen mask; and anticipate order to obtain arterial blood gases.

*Notes:*____

____

____

Fast facts in a nutshell: summary

You now have a strong foundation to assess and treat respiratory emergencies. Be sure to thoroughly document respiratory assessments, which should include rate, depth, breath sounds, symmetry, skin color, use of accessory muscles, if labored or unlabored, and ability to speak in full sentences. It is imperative that you are competent in recognizing and treating all respiratory emergencies. To make you more comfortable with respiratory problems, be sure to familiarize yourself with all your facility's respiratory supplies and equipment. Knowing where your supplies are and how to use them will make your job easier. If you have a lot of questions, a respiratory therapist can be a good resource. Never forget: in any emergency treat the airway first, then breathing, and then circulation.

Chapter 18

Shock and Multisystem Trauma Emergencies

INTRODUCTION

Patients in shock or with multisystem trauma are considered critical, *so a knowledge of these emergencies is vital for the emergency room nurse. The window of opportunity to save these patients' lives is small. In this chapter, you will learn the various forms of shock and how to intervene. You will also gain a better understanding of multiple types of trauma and how to manage them. Be sure to learn your facility's trauma protocols and be familiar with any trauma or shock supplies. It is also highly recommended that you sign up for and take the trauma nurse core course. It is a valuable certification to have and will help increase your knowledge in this area.*

During this part of your orientation, become familiar with and locate:

1. Rapid infusers, blood warmers, blood tubing, and blood bank.
2. Trauma protocols.
3. Drugs to know: dopamine, norepinephrine (Levophed), epinephrine, methylprednisolone sodium succinate (Solu-Medrol), dexamethasone (Decadron), diphenhydramine hydrochloride (Benadryl), and famotidine (Pepcid).
4. C-spine immobilization devices.
5. Anaphylactic drug supply box.

DIAGNOSES

Hemorrhagic/Hypovolemic Shock

This is a loss of too much blood volume. Hypovolemic shock is the most common form of shock in a trauma patient.

1. *Causes:* lack blood volume because of laceration of a major blood vessel; gastrointestinal bleeding; severe dehydration; ruptured organ; bleeding aneurysm; and poor clotting factors.
2. *Signs and symptoms:* hypotension; narrowing pulse pressure; tachycardia; and altered level of consciousness.
3. *Interventions:* treat airway, then breathing, and then circulation (ABCs); monitor vital signs, cardiac performance, and oxygen levels; anticipate orders to: obtain two large-bore intravenous accesses, administer IV crystalloid fluid infusion of 20 to 40 ml/kg, prepare transfusion of whole or packed red blood cells and fresh frozen plasma or platelets, and apply direct pressure to profusely bleeding lacerations.

Fast facts in a nutshell

Question: In a pediatric patient what are some late signs of hypovolemic shock?
Answer: *Bradycardia, hypotension. Cyanosis and tachycardia are early signs.*

Question: A patient with hyperosmolar hyperglycemic nonketotic syndrome is at risk for what type of shock?
Answer: *Hypovolemic shock.*

Question: Falling systolic pressure and rising diastolic pressure is indicative of what?
Answer: *Early shock class I.*

Question: What is the only intravenous fluid that can be infused with blood?
Answer: *Normal saline.*

Anaphylactic Shock

A systemic antigen-antibody response to an allergic reaction that is associated with sudden severe respiratory distress.

1. *Causes:* Unknown, but various triggers may stimulate a severe allergic reaction, including seafood; iodine; certain antibiotics; insect bites; nuts; and various medications or food.

2. *Signs and symptoms:* laryngeal edema; bronchospasms; wheezing; angioedema; and hypotension due to peripheral vasodilation.
3. *Interventions:* establish airway; apply oxygen; monitor cardiac performance; open intravenous access; obtain anaphylactic drug box; and administer medications (epinephrine, antihistamines, bronchodilators, and intravenous steroid) as ordered.

Notes: ______________________________________

____

____

Cardiogenic Shock

In cardiogenic shock, the heart fails to pump blood.

1. *Causes:* myocardial infarction; cardiac failure; or myocardial contusion.
2. *Signs and symptoms:* hypoxia; anxiety; diaphoretic and rapid weak pulse; arrhythmias; jugular vein distention; hypotension; pulmonary edema; and tachypnea.
3. *Interventions:* treat airway, then breathing, and then circulation (ABCs). Anticipate orders to: apply cardiac monitor, open two large-bore intravenous accesses, administer oxygen, take electrocardiogram and pulse oxygen, administer intravenous fluid bolus and administer appropriate antiarrhythmic medications, treat the underlying heart condition, and consider dobutamine.

*Notes:*____

____

____

Septic Shock

A systemic infection or severe sepsis. The very young, elderly, and immunosuppressed patients are more at risk.

1. *Causes:* typically due to gram-negative or gram-positive bacteria. The infection usually stems from one source and then spreads to the rest of the body through the bloodstream. A massive inflammatory response is launched by the body, which results in vasodilation and hypotension.
2. *Signs and symptoms:* fever early on; afebrile in late stage; confusion; hypotension; and weakness.
3. *Interventions:* look for underlying infection; monitor vital signs and temperature; anticipate orders to: start intravenous access, take blood cultures and a complete blood count, administer intravenous antibiotics, and obtain urine culture.

Fast facts in a nutshell

Question: Would you obtain blood cultures before or after administering intravenous antibiotics?
Answer: *Before x 2 from two different sites.*

*Notes:*____

____

____

Neurogenic Shock

This is the loss of sympathetic vasomotor regulation.

1. *Causes:* brain stem injury; spinal anesthesia; or spinal cord injury. Other causes may include drug use, such as tranquilizers; barbiturates; or anesthetics.
2. *Signs and symptoms:* peripheral vasodilation; neurological deficits; warm or flushed skin; and severe hypotension.
3. *Interventions:* provide airway, then breathing, and then circulation (ABCs); maintain cervical (C-spine) immobilization if spinal cord injury is present. Anticipate orders to: obtain intravenous access, administer intravenous fluid bolus, make neurological assessments, give dopamine or norepinephrine (Levophed), and reduce intracranial pressure.

*Notes:*____

____

____

Cardiothoracic Traumas

These traumas may be the result of motor vehicle collisions; gunshot wounds; falls; blasts; blows to the chest; or crushing injuries.

Pneumothorax: an air leak in the pleural space resulting in partial or total collapse of the lung.

1. *Causes:* A puncture to the lung due to chest trauma that results in an air leak.
2. *Signs and symptoms:* sucking chest wound; dyspnea; tachypnea; tachycardia; sudden pleuritic chest pain; anxiety; restlessness; diminished or absent breath sounds on affected side; pallor; hypotension if severe; subcutaneous emphysema; palpitations; or asymptomatic if small.
3. *Interventions:* put patient in high-Fowler's position; give oxygen; cover open chest wounds with flap Vaseline gauze dressing secured on three sides; anticipate orders to: check pulse oximetry, connect to cardiac monitor, arrange for immediate chest X-ray, prepare to assist with needle thoracostomy or chest tube insertion, administer pain meds, and obtain intravenous access.

*Notes:*____

____

____

Tension Pneumothorax: a life-threatening complication of pneumothorax.

1. *Causes:* The lung totally collapses and the heart and chest contents actually shift toward the unaffected lung.

2. *Signs and symptoms:* tracheal shift; severe respiratory distress; hypotension and jugular vein distention; dyspnea; tachypnea; tachycardia; sudden pleuritic chest pain; anxiety; restlessness; asymmetrical chest expansion; diminished or absent breath sounds on affected side; pallor; hypotension if severe; subcutaneous emphysema; and palpitations.
3. *Interventions:* treat airway, then breathing, and then circulation (ABCs); place in high-Fowler's position; anticipate orders to: prepare for needle thoracentesis and/or chest tube insertion, administer pain medications, arrange for chest X-ray, and apply sterile nonporous dressing (Vaseline gauze) with tape on three sides over an open-wound penetrating chest wound.

*Notes:*______________________________________

____

____

Hemothorax: blood leak in the pleural space resulting in partial or total collapse of the lung.

1. *Causes:* penetrating chest trauma with bleeding into the lung.
2. *Signs and symptoms:* If blood loss is greater than 1500 ml: mediastinal shift (systolic blood pressure of less than 80 mm Hg, and capillary refill of more than 4 sec); decreased urine output; respiratory distress; hypotension; cyanosis; tracheal deviation; decreased or absent breath sounds; and flat neck veins due to hypovolemic shock.
3. *Interventions:* treat airway, then breathing, and then circulation (ABCs); assist with chest tube insertion; antici-

pate orders to: prepare for emergency thoracotomy, open two large-bore intravenous accesses, administer intravenous fluid bolus, monitor cardiac performance, and prepare for emergency blood transfusion. If large volume of blood loss, anticipate autotransfusion.

*Notes:*____

____

____

Flail Chest: fracture of two or more ribs in two or more places resulting in a free-floating segment of the chest wall. Mortality increases if bilateral injury is present.

1. *Causes:* chest trauma.
2. *Signs and symptoms:* paradoxical chest movement; chest pain; dyspnea; tachypnea; and crepitus.
3. *Interventions:* treat airway, then breathing, and then circulation (ABCs); anticipate orders to: start intravenous access, monitor pulse oximetry, control pain, and prepare for possible intubation for ventilation assistance.

Fast facts in a nutshell

Question: What is the most serious injury associated with fractures of 1st and 2nd ribs?
Answer: *Aortic rupture.*

*Notes:*____________________________________

____

____

Cardiac Tamponade

This is fluid or blood build-up in pericardial sac surrounding the heart.

1. *Causes:* chest trauma. Also often found in penetrating chest trauma.
2. *Signs and symptoms:* penetrating chest wound noted to left 3rd to 5th ribs; muffled heart sounds; dyspnea; distended neck veins; facial cyanosis; hypotension; ST-segment elevation in all leads on electrocardiogram; chest wall ecchymosis; and elevated venous pressure.
3. *Interventions:* anticipate orders to: monitor cardiac performance, administer oxygen, open intravenous access, take electrocardiogram, and prepare for emergency pericardiocentesis.

Fast facts in a nutshell

Question: What autoimmune condition may cause cardiac tamponade?
Answer: *Systemic lupus erythematosus.*

*Notes:*____

____

____

Ruptured Diaphragm

A tear or rupture of the diaphragm; it can be a life-threatening injury.

1. *Causes:* blunt or penetrating forces resulting in herniation of abdominal contents into the thoracic cavity.
2. *Signs and symptoms:* epigastric pain; chest pain; abdominal pain; bowel sounds in lower chest; dyspnea; dysphagia; and decreased breath sounds.
3. *Interventions:* anticipate orders to: monitor cardiac performance and pulse oximetry, use nasogastric tube for stomach decompression, establish intravenous access, and prepare for surgery.

*Notes:*____

____

____

Spinal Cord Traumas

These traumas may result in spinal shock or neurogenic shock.

1. *Causes:* neck or back trauma.
2. *Signs and symptoms:* breathing difficulty; varying paralysis depending on injury location; bradycardia; hypotension; autonomic dysreflexia (hypertensive condition: headache, sweating, and bradycardia); warm and dry skin; may assume room temperature; pain; and possible priapism.
3. *Interventions:* open airway maintaining cervical (C-spine) immobilization (use jaw thrust-chin lift maneuver); conduct a neurological assessment; logroll the patient when turning; prepare for possible endotracheal intubation; assist if ventilation assistance required; anticipate orders to: administer intravenous fluids and steroids, insert nasogastric tube and Foley catheter, provide warming measures for hypothermia, and take measures to avoid skin breakdown.

Fast facts in a nutshell

Question: Children younger than eight years of age are most likely to have what type of spinal cord injury?
Answer: *Cervical spine C1–C3.*

Notes:

Abdominal Traumas

Splenic Injuries: trauma or injury to the spleen.

1. *Causes:* usually occurs with blunt left upper quadrant abdominal trauma.
2. *Signs and symptoms:* Kehr's sign (left upper quadrant abdominal pain that may radiate to the left shoulder); absent or hypoactive bowel sounds; abdominal muscle rigidity; and hypovolemic shock.
3. *Interventions:* abdominal assessment (look, listen, and feel); anticipate orders to: establish large-bore intravenous access, administer intravenous fluids, type and screen blood, and prepare for blood transfusion and surgical intervention.

> **Fast facts in a nutshell**
>
> **Question:** In blunt abdominal trauma, which organ is most commonly injured?
> **Answer:** *The spleen.*

The highly vascular ruptured spleen is a life-threatening injury. Check Kehr's sign (see Figure 18.1), which is a sharp pain radiating to the left scapula.

Notes: ______________________________

____

____

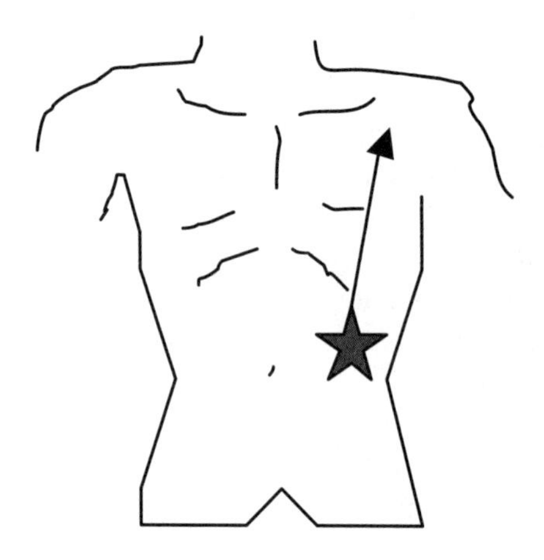

Figure 18.1

Pelvic Fractures: either stable or unstable. With a pelvic fracture, your patient can lose up to about 3000 ml of blood!

1. *Causes:* pelvic trauma.
2. *Signs and symptoms:* pain; pelvic instability; rigidity; hypoactive bowel sounds; hypovolemic shock; and leg shortening or rotation. If urethral laceration: blood from urethral meatus. If bladder laceration: suprapubic pain and an inability to void.
3. *Interventions:* anticipate orders to: apply antishock trousers, establish large-bore intravenous access, administer intravenous isotonic fluid bolus, arrange for pelvic X-ray or CT scan, type and screen blood, and prepare for possible surgery.

Fast facts in a nutshell

Question: What are some uses for pneumatic anti-shock garment?
Answer: *Unstable pelvic fractures, bilateral femur fractures, abdominal trauma, and retroperitoneal hemorrhage.*

Notes: ____________________

____

____

Head Traumas

Linear Skull Fracture: a nondepressed skull fracture.

1. *Causes:* head trauma.
2. *Signs and symptoms:* pain over fracture; scalp laceration; headache; and possible decreased level of consciousness.
3. *Interventions:* obtain neurological assessment; clean and dress any wounds; arrange for skull X-rays or head CT scans; and follow head injury patient teaching instructions upon discharge.

Notes: ____________________

____

____

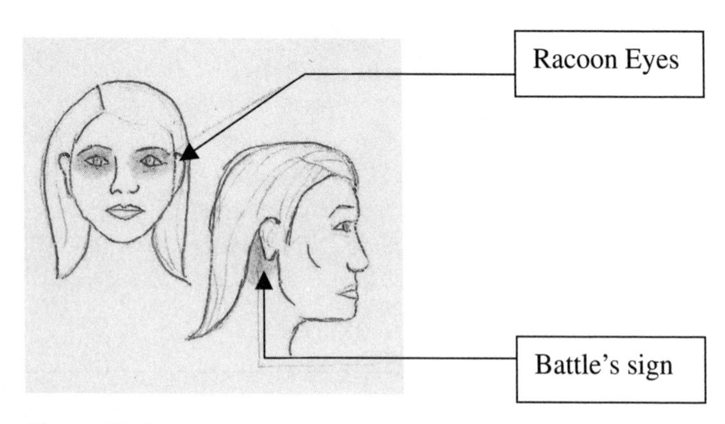

Figure 18.2

Basilar Skull Fracture: a fracture to the bones at the base of the skull. Complications include infection and cerebrospinal fluid leak.

1. *Causes:* head trauma to base of skull.
2. *Signs and symptoms:* altered level of consciousness; bruising behind the ear (Battle's sign) 12 to 24 hours after injury; bruising around the eyes (Racoon's eyes) 12 to 24 hours after injury; headache; rhinorrhea; otorrhea; and unilateral hearing loss. See Figure 18.2.
3. *Interventions:* If there is a cerebral spinal fluid leak, apply dry sterile loose dressing below the drainage. Obtain neurological assessments; anticipate orders to: arrange for X-rays and head CT scan, establish intravenous access, administer antibiotics, and prepare oral gastric tube for gastric decompression.

*Notes:*____

____

____

____

Depressed Skull Fracture: a concave-like skull fracture.

1. *Causes:* direct blow to the head; head trauma.
2. *Signs and symptoms:* altered level of consciousness; head laceration; headache; and skull depression noted upon palpation.
3. *Interventions:* apply loose sterile dressing; perform neurological assessment; anticipate orders to: establish intravenous access, administer antibiotics, arrange for X-rays and head CT scan.

> **Fast facts in a nutshell**
>
> A loose sterile dressing is used on a depressed skull fracture and nasal cerebral spinal fluid leaks.

*Notes:*____

____

____

____

Concussion: a closed head injury resulting in transient neurological changes.

1. *Causes:* head trauma
2. *Signs and symptoms:* nausea; vomiting; dizziness; headache; altered level of consciousness; seizure; poor balance; and possible amnesia.
3. *Interventions:* perform a neurological assessment; elevate head of bed; anticipate orders for: head CT scan and hospital admission if loss of consciousness lasts more than 5 minutes or patient remains confused, and provide head injury discharge instructions.

*Notes:*____

____

____

Subdural Hematoma: bleeding between the dura mater (outermost brain covering) and the arachnoid layer (fine fibrous layer between dura and pia mater) of meninges resulting in direct pressure of brain surface.

1. *Causes:* commonly caused by head trauma or violent shaking.
2. *Signs and symptoms:* loss of consciousness; deteriorating mental status; fixed and dilated pupil on side of injury; increased intracranial pressure; immediate and prolonged coma; and posturing (dec**or**ticate, toward the **cord**; decerebrate, away from the cord). See Figure 18.3.
3. *Interventions:* perform neurological assessment; anticipate orders for: a head CT scan, measures to reduce intracranial pressure, and prepare patient for neurosurgery.

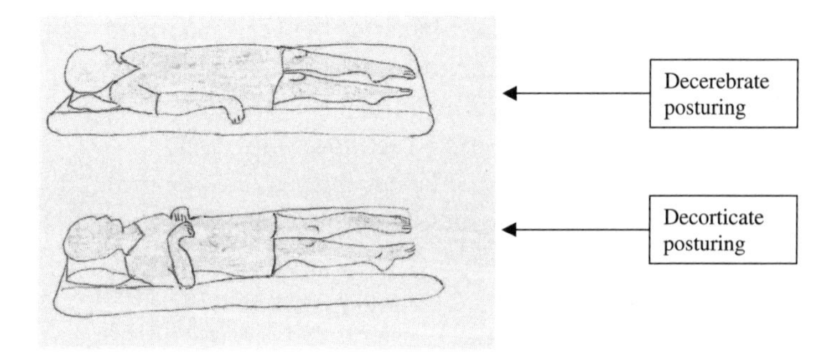

Figure 18.3

*Notes:*____

____

____

Epidural Hematoma: bleeding between skull and dura mater.

1. *Causes:* head trauma. It commonly occurs with temporal and parietal skull fractures.
2. *Signs and symptoms:* loss of consciousness; ipsilateral pupil dilation; posturing; and hemiparesis.
3. *Interventions:* perform neurological assessment; anticipate orders for: a head CT scan, measures to reduce intracranial pressure, and prepare patient for surgery.

*Notes:*____

____

____

Subarachnoid Hemorrhage: bleeding between pia mater (delicate surface layer of brain) and arachnoid membrane.

1. *Causes:* head trauma. This injury is frequently associated with child abuse and has a high mortality rate.
2. *Signs and symptoms:* headache; nausea and vomiting; altered level of consciousness; neurological deficits; seizure; and posturing.
3. *Interventions:* prepare neurological assessment; anticipate order to arrange for head CT scan; and prepare for surgery.

*Notes:*____

____

____

Contusion: bruise to the brain surface.

1. *Causes:* direct blow to the head.
2. *Signs and symptoms:* neurological deficits; altered level of consciousness; nausea and vomiting; amnesia; seizure; and posturing.
3. *Interventions:* perform neurological assessment; arrange for head CT scan when ordered; and provide head injury patient teaching upon discharge.

*Notes:*____

____

____

Increased Intracranial Pressure

1. *Causes:* head trauma, electrolyte imbalances, and meningitis.
2. *Signs and symptoms:* altered level of consciousness; oval-shaped pupil; Cheyne-Stokes respirations; and bulging fontanels in children younger than two years of age.
3. *Interventions:* anticipate orders to: administer mannitol, hyperventilate patient, elevate head of bed to 30°, and avoid Valsalva maneuver.

Notes: ____

____

____

Fast facts in a nutshell: summary

You now have a stronger knowledge base for shock and multisystem emergencies. Shock and trauma emergencies are always critical situations. You should be able to differentiate among the various types of shock and trauma and know how to respond. Finding time to chart during a critical emergency is difficult. Most of the time, you need another nurse to help. All emergency room nurses have to be team players. Even still, you may have to jot your notes on a scratch piece of paper and document later. To ease any anxiety, take some deep and cleansing breaths, get help, and learn as much as you can about shock and trauma.

Chapter 19

Substance Abuse and Toxicologic Emergencies

INTRODUCTION

Substance abuse and toxicologic conditions, which are seen regularly in the emergency room, can be fatal. Because so many types of substance abuse and poisonous materials exist, remembering them all is difficult. However, never fear. This chapter will provide a simple and easy-to-use substance abuse and toxicology table. Even with access to this table, you must still always consult with poison control after the patient is triaged. Poison control will give you vital individualized suggestions based on the patient's weight, circumstances, amount of drug intake, and the time frame in which the drug was taken. Document and communicate the suggestions provided by poison control with the emergency room provider to obtain any necessary immediate orders.

During this part of your orientation, locate and become familiar with:

1. Local poison control number.
2. Drugs to know: charcoal with or without sorbitol, naloxone (Narcan), flumazenil (Romazicon), acetylcysteine (Mucomyst), and banana bag.
3. Your local poisonous snakes and appropriate antivenom information.
4. Nasogastric tubes and gastric lavage equipment.

Fast facts in a nutshell

- Call poison control for *EVERY* overdose.
- Treatment of most overdose patients generally begins with the ABCs (Airway, Breathing, Circulation) and MOVE (Monitor, Oxygen, Venous access, and Electrocardiogram).

Table 19.1 is a great quick reference tool to assist you with substance abuse and toxicology cases. In it, you will find an alphabetical list of each substance or drug class, with the corresponding symptoms and interventions. Examples of drugs and substances are provided under each class.

*Notes:*____

____

____

Fast facts in a nutshell

Question: Why can't you rely on a pulse oxygen reading in carbon monoxide poisoning?
Answer: *Carbon dioxoide, ethane, methane, propane, and other fuel gases don't react or bind to hemoglobin. Therefore, you can not rely on pulse oxygen reading. Treatment is "fresh air" or supplemental oxygen.*

Question: Ecstasy use along with increased water intake to avoid hyperthermia can lead to what electrolyte imbalance?
Answer: *Hyponatremia.*

Question: A college student arrives in the emergency room complaining of palpitations and chest pain. He admits to using cocaine. What should you suspect?
Answer: *Acute myocardial infarction.*

Question: How does charcoal leave the digestive system?
Answer: *Usually it comes out in the form of black diarrhea. An unconscious or confused patient may need an incontinence pad.*

TABLE 19.1 Substance Abuse and Toxicology Table

Drug/Substance	Signs and Symptoms	Interventions/anticipated orders
Acetylcholinesterase Inhibition (Cholinergics): insecticides, organophosphates, carbamates, and nerve agents	*remember SLUDGE* **S**aliva, **L**acrimation, **U**rination, **D**efecation, **G**I upset, and **E**mesis. Early on tachycardia; lethargic; paralysis; shock; anxiety; bronchospasms; ataxia; pulmonary edema; bradypnea; seizure; and coma. Bradycardia in late stages.	Wash toxins off the patient. If oral ingestion, give 1 gm/kg charcoal. Atropine may reverse central nervous system effects. Ipratropium bromide (Atrovent) nebulized treatment may dry secretions. Administer pralidoxime or obidoxime.
Alcohol Abuse: liquors, beers, wines, moonshine, rubbing alcohol, even mouthwash.	Slurred speech; unsteady gait; and alcohol odor. The patient may go into withdrawal.	Obtain alcohol level. Intravenous banana bag and time for alcohol levels to drop. Lorazepam (Ativan) helps with withdrawal.

Anticholinergic Overdose: dicyclomine, tropicamide, alkaloids cyclopentolate, homatropine, phenothiazines, amanita muscarina, jimson-weed or deadly nightshade, belladonna, atropine, and tricyclics.	Hallucinations; delirium; blurred vision; tachycardia; arrhythmias; fever; abdominal distention; urine retention; ataxia; cardio-vascular collapse; seizure; hypertension; thirst; hot/flushed/dry skin; dilated pupils; and mydriasis.	Physostigmine and 1 gm/kg charcoal if ingestion was less than one hour ago.
Benzodiazepines: Serax, Rohypnol aka "roofies" are 10× as potent as diazepam	Drowsiness; confusion; bradypnea; sedation; and hypotension.	Administer flumazenil (Romazicon)
Beta Blockers: atenolol, metoprolol, propranolol, and sotalol.	Bradycardia; hypotension; shock; and cardiac arrest.	Administer 1–5 mg gluconate intravenously/intramuscularly/subcutaneously. Give intra-venous normal saline bolus for hypotension; and prepare pace-maker and calcium IV push.
Calcium Channel Blockers: verapamil, nifedipine (Procardia), and diltiazem	Bradycardia; hypotension; lethargy; confusion; bradypnea; nausea and vomiting; shock; hyper-glycemia; and cardiac arrest	1 Gm calcium gluconate intra-venously over five minutes until response seen or maximum of 4 Gm. Give normal saline bolus.

(continued)

TABLE 19.1 *(Continued)*

Drug/Substance	Signs and Symptoms	Interventions/anticipated orders
Carbon Monoxide Poisoning: carbon monoxide displaces oxygen on the hemoglobin	Hypoxia; confusion; headache; nausea and vomiting; dizziness; coma; seizures; cyanosis; and death.	Give oxygen via nonrebreather mask; provide hyperbaric oxygen treatment; and obtain carbon dioxide levels.
Cardiac Glycosides: digoxin, digitoxin, oleander, and foxglove.	Visual-yellow green halos; nausea and vomiting; headache; bradycardia; ventricular arrhythmias; shock; and cardiac arrest.	Obtain digoxin level; give Digibind (digoxin) immune fab; administer 1 Gm/kg charcoal and 1 mg/kg lidocaine intravenously for arrhythmias, and give atropine.
Ethylene Glycol (antifreeze)	*First 1–12 hours:* slurred speech; inebriated; coma; seizure; and death. *12–24 hrs:* tachycardia; hypertension; tachypnea; congestive heart failure; acute respiratory distress syndrome; and cardiac collapse.	Labs: determine serum ethylene glycol level; prepare basic metabolic panel; and obtain urinalysis. Give gastric lavage (charcoal is ineffective), 50 mEq IV sodium bicarb; 10% 10–20 ml calcium gluconate intravenously, 2 g IV mag-

	24–72 hrs: nephrotoxicity; flank pain; renal failure; and hypocalcemia.	nesium; 100 mg intravenous thiamine; 15 mg/kg intravenous fomepizole (Antizol); and prepare for dialysis.
Hallucinogens: LSD (D-Lysergic Acid diethylamide) abuse.	Agitation; hallucinations; dilated pupils; hyperthemic; and tachycardia.	Reassure and reorient to reality; instruct patient to keep eyes open; and provide good lighting to decrease shadows. Give benzodiazepines for agitation.
Heparin	Bleeding	Obtain partial thromboplastin time level and give protamine sulfate.
Insulin	Weak; lethargic; syncope; and blood sugar less than 80.	Monitor blood sugar; give 1 amp dextrose (D_{50}) intravenously or feed the patient a meal. Give 5–10 mg glucagon IV over 1 minute.
Nonspecific or unknown	Varies	Activated charcoal in water or 1 Gm/kg sorbitol.

(continued)

TABLE 19.1 *(Continued)*

Drug/Substance	Signs and Symptoms	Interventions/anticipated orders
Narcotics (Opioids): morphine, methadone, dextromethorphan, heroin, fentanyl, meperidine (Demerol), codeine, diphenoxylate and propoxyphene.	Pinpoint pupils (miosis); central nervous system depression; depression; bradycardia; hypotension; and bradypnea.	Intravenous 0.4–2 mg Narcan every 2–3 minutes up to 10 mg.
Salicylates: aspirin	Nausea and vomiting; tinnitus; diaphoresis; acidosis; altered mental status; seizures; and shock.	Dialysis and 1 mEq/kg sodium bicarbonate intravenously.
Stimulants (Sympathomimetics): aminophylline, amphetamines, cocaine, ephedrine, caffeine, methylphenidates, methamphetamines, and PCP	Hypertension; dilated pupils; tachycardia; paranoia; vasoconstriction; hyperthermia; seizures; chest pain; acute myocardial infarction; coma (hypotension with caffeine); and altered mood.	Give benzodiazepines, nitroglycerin or nitroprusside (Nipride) for hypertension, haloperidol (Haldol), and 1 Gm/kg charcoal.

Tricyclic Antidepressants: amitriptyline, desipramine, nortriptyline, and imipramine.	Tachycardia; bradycardia; ventricular arrhythmias; shock; and cardiac arrest.	1 mEq per kg IV sodium bicarb for tricyclic antidepressants to obtain serum pH of 7.50–7.55 to alter protein binding; give normal saline bolus; hyperventile; give norepinephrine (Levophed) if hypotension; and give magnesium sulfate.
Tylenol Overdose: can lead to liver failure and death. 140 mg/kg is toxic	*First 24 hrs:* asymptomatic; minor gastrointestinal upset. *24–72 hrs:* elevated liver function test or renal failure. *72–96 hrs:* jaundice; renal failure; coagulopathy; and liver necrosis. *4 days–2 wks:* symptoms resolve or patient dies.	Labs: acetaminophen level 4 hours after ingestion. Administer Mucomyst (acetylcysteine) the sooner the better. May be useful up to 72 hours after ingestion.
Venom of Rattlesnakes, Cottonmouths, and Copperheads	Bite/fang marks with redness/bruising; pain; and swelling.	Antivenin, crotalidae polyvalent (CroFab) 3–5 vials in 250–500 mg normal saline for mild symptoms.
Warfarin (Coumadin)	Bleeding	Obtain prothrombin time and INR level, and give vitamin K.

Fast facts in a nutshell: summary

You now have a stronger knowledge base for substance abuse and toxicology emergencies. You should able to differentiate the types of substance abuse and toxicology emergencies and know how to respond. It is vital to obtain the best history possible from your patient. Because your patient may not be responsive, speak with any witnesses, friends, or family. Each overdose case is different. Many factors will affect the treatment, including time of ingestion, amount of substance, patient's weight, and current vital signs. Be sure to contact poison control for every case. They will help you and the provider come up with the proper individualized treatment course needed.

Appendices

Appendix A

Common Emergency Room Lab Values

Lab	Normal value	High value causes	Low value causes
Glucose	70–110	Diabetic ketoacidosis; hyperglycemic nonketotic coma	Insulin overdose
Creatinine	0.6–1.3	Renal disease	
Blood urea nitrogen (BUN)	7–18	Renal disease	
Sodium (Na)	135–145	Sweating, diarrhea, diabetes	Congestive heart failure; cirrhosis; renal failure; nausea, vomiting, and diarrhea; excess water intake

(continued)

Lab	Normal value	High value causes	Low value causes
Potassium (K)	3.5–5.1	Metabolic acidosis	Poor potassium intake; diuretics; nausea, vomiting, and diarrhea
CO_2	21–32	Respiratory acidosis	
Aspartate aminotrans-ferase/serum glutamic-oxaloacetic transaminase (AST/SGOT)	15–37	Liver damage	
Alanine aminotrans-ferase/serum glutamic pyruvic transaminase (ALT/SGPT)	30–65	Liver damage	
Lipase	114–286	Pancreatitis; cholecystitis	
Amylase	25–115	Pancreatitis; cholecystitis	
White blood cell count (WBC)	4–11	Infection; inflammation; leukemia—very high levels	Neutropenia

Lab	Normal value	High value causes	Low value causes
Red blood cell count (RBC)	4.2–5.5	Dehydration	Anemia
Hemoglobin (HGB)	12–16	Dehydration	Anemia; gastrointestinal bleeding
Hematocrit (HCT)	37–47	Dehydration	Anemia; gastro-intestinal bleeding
Platelets (PLT)	140–440	Chronic inflammation	Thrombocyto-penia
Troponin	0–0.10	Myocardial infarction	
Creatine kinase-MB (CKMB)	0–3.6	Myocardial infarction	
D-dimer	0–682	Congestive heart failure; pulmonary embolism	
Partial thrombo-plastin time (PTT)	18–41 Varies	Hemophilia; heparin overdose; disseminated intravascular coagulation (DIC)	

(continued)

Lab	Normal value	High value causes	Low value causes
Prothrombin time (PT)	11–14 (varies)	Coumadin overdose; decreased potassium; liver disease	
Calcium (Ca)	8.5–10.6	Hyperthyroidism; tuberculosis; too much vitamin D	Pancreatitis; parathyroid trauma; alcohol abuse; renal failure

Appendix B

Everyday Emergency Room Medications*

Medication	Dose	Use
Acetaminophen (Tylenol, Datril)	Adult: 500–1,000 mg Child: 15 mg/kg	Fever and pain.
Acetaminophen with codeine (Tylenol with Codeine)	Doses vary. Codeine component of 15–60 mg. Tylenol dose is 300–1,000 mg. Every 4 hours PO.	Analgesic.
Acetylcysteine (Mucomyst)	Adult/child: PO 140 mg/kg, then 70 mg/kg every 4 hours. Intravenous loading: 150 mg/kg over 60 min	Antidote for Tylenol overdose.

(continued)

*The definitions of abbreviations can be found in Appendix D.

Medication	Dose	Use
Acetylsalicylic acid (Aspirin)	160–325 mg by mouth or by rectum.	CP-blood thinner.
Adenosine (Adenocard)	Initial intravenous bolus 6 mg rapidly over 1–3 sec. Follow with normal saline bolus. 2nd or 3rd dose of 12 mg rapid intravenous push	Narrow complex PSVT or SVT. NOT for A-fib, A-flutter, or VT.
Albuterol (Proventil)	Child: MDI 0.1 mg/kg (max 2.5) three times a day. Neb 0.1–0.15 mg/kg/dose four times a day. Adult: 2 puffs of metered dose inhaler every 4 hours, Neb 2.5 mg four times a day.	Bronchodilator for asthma/chronic obstructive pulmonary disease. Also treat hyperkalemia.
Amiodarone hydrochloride (Cordarone, Pacerone)	Load 150 mg over 10 min, then 360 mg over 6 hours intravenously.	Life-threatening ventricular arrhythmias.
Atenolol (Tenormin)	5 mg intravenous over 5 min, wait 10 min, may give a second 5 mg. Wait 10 min then 50 mg by mouth.	Acute myocardial infarction; supraventricular tachycardia; PSVT, A-fib, A-flutter, antihypertensive.

Medication	Dose	Use
Atropine sulfate (Atropen)	Intravenous push: 1 mg every 3–5 min. Maximum of 3 mg. ET: 2–3 mg in 10 ml normal saline.	Asystole, pulseless electrical activity, bradycardia, and organophosphate poisoning.
Azithromycin (Zithromax)	Adult: By mouth 500 mg 1st dose then 250 mg every day for four days. For gonorrhea 1–2 Gm by mouth × 1 dose. Intravenous: 500 mg/hr every day.	Antibiotic used commonly for gonorrhea; PID; and respiratory infections.
Banana Bag: (1 L D_5 NS, 1 mg folic acid, 1 amp MVI, and 100 mg thiamine). You can add 1–3 Gm magnesium sulfate	250 ml/hr intravenous	Chronic alcohol abuse and malnourishment.
Calcium chloride	500–1,000 mg intravenous. Do NOT mix with bicarbonate.	Hyperkalemia, calcium channel or beta blocker overdose, hypocalcemia.

(continued)

Medication	Dose	Use
Ceftriaxone sodium (Rocephin) *can mix with lidocaine 1% as directed on box*	Adult: 250 mg–2 G intravenous/IM per day. Child: 25–50 mg/kg/every 12 hours.	Antibiotic for infection.
Charcoal in water. No sorbitol for a child due to diarrhea/ dehydration	Child/Adult 1 Gm/kg by mouth	Antidote for toxins. Can mix with chocolate syrup, coke, or fruit juice for children.
Charcoal with Sorbitol	Adult: 1 Gm/kg by mouth	Antidote for toxins.
D50, Glucose (Dextrose)	Average dose 0.5–1 amp intravenous. Check blood sugar.	Acute hypoglycemia.
Diazepam (Valium). Do NOT mix with anything	Intravenous: 2–20 mg. Per rectum: 0.2–0.5 mg/ kg max 20 mg.	Seizures and sedation.
Digoxin (Lanoxin)	Loading: 10–15 mg/kg.	A-fib, A-flutter, or SVT.

Medication	Dose	Use
Digoxin immune Fab (Digibind)	Varies depending on digoxin level, with an average 400–800 mg	Digoxin overdose; digitalis toxicity.
Diltiazem hydrochloride (Cardizem)	15–20 mg (0.25 mg/kg) intravenous over 2 min. May repeat in 15 min at 0.35 mg/kg. Infuse at 5–15 mg/h	A-fib or A-flutter.
Dobutamine hydrochloride (Dobutrex) 250 mg in 250 ml D_5W (1 mg/ml)	2–20 mcg/kg/min intravenous drip.	Vasopressor. Pump problems: congestive heart failure without symptoms of shock.
Dopamine hydrochloride (Intropin) 400 mg in 250 ml D_5W (1,600 mcg/ml)	2–20 mcg/kg/min intravenous drip	Vasopressor for hypotension and shock.
Enalapril maleate (Vasotec)	1.25–5 mg intravenous over 5 min.	Hypertension.

(continued)

Medication	Dose	Use
Enoxaparin sodium (Lovenox)	1 mg/kg twice daily. Subcutaneously in abdomen only	Myocardial infarction–anticoagulant.
Epinephrine 1:10,000 intravenous or 1:1000 for subcutaneous administration.	Intravenously: 1 mg/10 ml of 1:10,000 solution every 3–5 min. ET: 2–2.5 mg in 10 ml normal saline. Subcutaneously: 0.1–0.5 of 1:1000 solution, may repeat in 20 min.	PEA, asystole, pulseless VT, V-fib, symptomatic bradycardia, anaphylaxis, and hypotension.
Etomidate (Amidate)	0.3–0.4 mg/kg intravenous	Sedation for intubation/shoulder reduction.
Flumazenil (Romazicon)	0.2–5.0 mg intravenously	Antidote for benzodiazepine overdose.
Fosphenytoin sodium (Cerebyx)	Load 15–20 phenytoin equivalents per kg by intramuscular injection or intravenous 150 mg/min or less	Seizures.
Furosemide (Lasix)	Intravenous 0.5–2 mg/kg over 1–2 min	Congestive heart failure, hypertension, intracranial pressure.

Medication	Dose	Use
Gentamicin sulfate ophthalmic ointment	0.5-inch ribbon to inside affected lower eyelid.	Conjunctivitis and corneal abrasions.
Glucagon	1 mg subcutaneous/ injection/intravenous push, followed by infusion of 3 mg/hr. Subcutaneously/by injection: 1 mg	Hypoglycemia, calcium channel or beta blocker overdose, and esophageal food bolus.
Haloperidol decanoate (Haldol)	Adult: 0.5–5 mg three times a day by mouth or injection	Antipsychotic.
Heparin sodium *check PTT & guaiac stool before giving	Intravenous bolus: 60 unit/kg max 4000 units. Then 12 unit/ kg/hr drip	Anticoagulant for acute myocardial infarction and stroke.
Hydrocodone bitartrate and acetamino-phen (Lortab)	Adult: 2.5–10 mg every 3–6 hours	Opioid analgesic for pain.
Ibuprofen (Motrin, Advil)	10 mg/kg by mouth, maximum of 800 mg	Pain or fever.

(continued)

Medication	Dose	Use
Insulin (Regular) *check blood sugar every hour*	Adult intravenous: 5–10 unit bolus, then intravenous drip 2–12 unit/h. Subcutaneously: 0.5–1 unit/kg/day	Diabetic ketoacidosis; hyperglycemia.
Ipratropium bromide (Atrovent)	Child: 125–250 mcg by nebulizer every 4–6 hours. Adult: 250–500 mcg by nebulizer four times a day. Maximum: 24 doses in 24 hours.	Bronchodilator/ anticholinergic for asthma and chronic obstructive pulmonary disease.
Labetalol hydrochloride (Normodyne)	0.25 mg/kg intravenous, may double dose every 10–15 min as often as necessary; maximum of 300 or 2 mg/kg.	Hypertension.
Levalbuterol hydrochloride (Xopenex)	Adult: 0.63–1.25 mg Neb. Child 6–12 yrs 0.31–0.63 mg Neb.	Bronchodilator for asthma. Causes less tachycardia than albuterol.
Levofloxacin (Levaquin) *if given too fast = arrhythmias*	500–750 mg by mouth/ intravenous drip at 500 mg/hr or 750 mg over 1.5 hr	Antibiotic.

Medication	Dose	Use
Lidocaine hydrochloride (Xylocaine)	Intravenous push: 1–1.5 mg/kg, may repeat at 0.5–0.75 mg/kg in 5–10 min. Intravenous drip 1–4 mg/min. ET: 2–4 mg/kg.	Ventricular fibrillation/ventricular tachycardia. Can be given subcutaneously locally to numb a wound. Comes in 1 or 2% vials.
Lidocaine with epinephrine *Not for finger/nose/ears/toes	Subcutaneously locally 1 or 2% vials	To numb a bleeding wound.
Lorazepam (Ativan)	0.1 mg/kg up to 4 mg intravenous or by injection.	Seizures and sedation.
Magnesium sulfate	Cardiac arrest: 1–2 g in 10 ml D_5W over 5–20 min. If stable: 1g/50 ml normal saline over 30 min intravenously.	Torsades de pointes, hypomagnesemia, and asthma: smooth muscle relaxant.
Mannitol strengths: 5, 10, 15, 20, and 25%	0.5–1 g/kg over 5–10 min use inline filter	Intracranial pressure.

(continued)

Medication	Dose	Use
Methotrexate	Adult: 50 mg/m^2 by IM	Miscarriages/ectopic pregnancy.
Meperidine hydrochloride (Demerol)	Adult: 25–100 mg by mouth/injection/ intravenous (average dose 25–75 mg).	Opioid analgesic.
Methyl-prednisolone (Solu-Medrol)	Adult 100–250 mg intravenous/by injection (average 125 mg)	Steroid to decrease inflammation in asthma; allergic reaction; shock.
Morphine sulfate	2–8 mg intravenously over 1–5 min	Chest pain or pain.
Naloxone hydrochloride (Narcan)	Intravenous: 0.4–2 mg max 10 mg in 10 min. By mouth or subcuta-neously: 0.4–0.8 mg. Can give via ET tube.	Opiate overdose with resp or neurodepression.
Nitroglycerin (Nitro-Dur, Nitrostat) *monitor blood pres-sure for hypo-tension; must have intra-venous access before giving.	Intravenous drip 10–20 mcg/min titrate for chest pain/blood pressure by 5–10 mcg/ min every 5–10 min. Under the tongue: 1 tab every 5 min for a 3 tablet maximum per blood pressure/chest pain	Vasodilator; chest pain; acute myocardial infarction; congestive heart failure; and hypertension.

Medication	Dose	Use
Nitroprusside sodium (Nipride) *med reacts to light; cover material provided from pharmacy.	Intravenous 0.1 mcg/kg/min titrate up every 5–10 minutes until stable blood pressure/chest pain; average dose 5–10 mcg/kg/min.	Hypertension; reduce afterload in congestive heart failure; pulmonary edema; or valve regurgitation.
Norepinephrine bitartrate (Levophed)	Adult: 2–4 mcg/min intravenous drip titrate to BP. Max 30 mcg/min.	Vasopressor for severe cardiogenic shock, drug overdose, or poison-induced hypotension.
Oxycodone and Acetaminophen (Percocet)	PO: 5–10 mg	Narcotic for pain.
Phenytoin sodium (Dilantin) *Infiltration = tissue necrosis, be careful.	20 mg/kg up to 1,000 mg intravenous. NO faster than 50 mg/min	Seizures. * Only mixes with normal saline.
Promethazine hydrochloride (Phenergan)	12.5–25 mg by mouth/injection/intravenous/suppository	Nausea and vomiting.

(continued)

Medication	Dose	Use
Proparacaine hydrochloride (Alcaine)	2–3 drops to affected eye.	To numb the eye. *If used repeatedly, can be corrosive to eye!*
Propranolol hydrochloride (Inderal)	Adult: 10–30 mg by mouth four times a day. Intravenous bolus: 0.5–3 mg at 1 mg/min, may repeat in 2 min.	Hypertension; acute myocardial infarction; dysrhythmias.
Reteplase, recombinant (Retavase) (*Perform checklist prior to administration)	1st dose: 10 unit intravenous bolus over 2 min. 2nd dose 30 min later 10 units intravenous bolus over 2 min	Clot buster for stroke or acute myocardial infarction.
RhoGAM injection	Adult: 300 mcg by injection	Rh-negative pregnant mother.
Sodium bicarbonate	Intravenous bolus: 1 mEq/kg	Acidosis; hyperkalemia; diabetic ketoacidosis; cocaine abuse, diphenhydramine or tricyclic antidepressant overdose.
Sodium polystyrene sulfonate (Kayexalate)	15–60 Gm by mouth.	Removes potassium from body.

Medication	Dose	Use
Succinyl-choline (Anectine)	0.6–1.5 mg/kg intravenous	Paralytic for intubation. Have ambu bag ready!
Tenecteplase (TNKase)	Intravenous bolus of 30–50 mg based on weight.	Fibrinolytic agent (clot buster) for acute myocardial infarction or ischemic stroke.
Tetracaine eyedrops	2–3 drops to affected eye	Topical anesthetic to the eye. *Repeated use = eye corrosion!
Vasopressin (Pitressin) *alternative to Epine-phrine	Intravenous/intraosseous push: 40 units Instead of 1st or 2nd dose of epinephrine	Cardiac arrest, V-fib, pulseless electrical activity, and asystole.
Verapamil hydrochloride	Intravenous bolus: 2.5–5 mg over 2 min. May repeat at 5–10 mg every 15–30 min. Max: 20 mg	PSVT with narrow complex. A-fib or A-flutter.
Warfarin sodium (Coumadin)	Adult: 2–10 mg/day.	Anticoagulant.

Data from Handbook, 2005; Rothrock, 2005; and Skidmore-Roth, 2009.

Appendix C

List of Important ER Medications

Fill out formulary kept in your hospital and keep this list taped to the back of your calculator:

Levophed: ____ mg/ ____ L (____ mcg/ml) give 2–4 mcg/min. max: 30
Dopamine: ____ mg/ ____ ml (____ mcg/ml) give 2–10 mcg/kg/min. max: 50
Diprivan: ____ mcg/ml give 5–10 mcg/kg/min
Lidocaine: ____ G/____ ml (____ mcg/ml) give 20–50 mcg/kg/min
Heparin ____ units/____ ml (____ units/ml) 1000 u/h
Nitroglycerin ____ mg/ ____ ml (____ mcg/ml) give 5–20 mcg/min
Dobutamine ____ mg/ ____ ml (____ mcg/ml) give 2.5–10 mcg/kg/min. max: 40
Nipride ____ mg/ ____ ml (____ mcg/ml) give 0.3–8 mcg/kg/min. max: 10
Amiodarone loading 150 mg over 10 min then 360 mg over 6 hr.

Appendix D

Abbreviations

The emergency room nurse must be familiar with many abbreviations. They allow for quicker oral and written communication. For the sake of clarity and readability, terms have been spelled out in the text. Common abbreviations for terms used in the text are listed below.

abd	abdominal
ABG	arterial blood gas
ACLS	advanced cardiovascular life support
ADH	antidiuretic hormone
A fib	atrial fibrillation
A flutter	atrial flutter
AIDS	acquired immunodeficiency syndrome
ALT/SGPT	alanine aminotransferase/serum glutamic pyruvic transaminase
AMI	acute myocardial infarct
ASAP	as soon as possible
AST/SGOT	aspartate aminotransferase/serum glutamic-oxaloacetic transaminase
ASD	atrial septal defect

AV	atrioventricular
AVSD	atrioventricular septal defect
b.i.d.	twice daily
BiPAP	bilevel positive airway pressure
BMP	basic metabolic panel
BP	blood pressure
bpm	beats per minute
BRAT	bananas, rice, applesauce, and toast
BS	blood sugar
BSC	bedside commode
BUN	blood urea nitrogen
BVM	bag valve mask
CAD	coronary artery disease
CBC	complete blood count
CDC	Centers for Disease Control
CHD	congenital heart disease
CHF	congestive heart failure
CKMB	creatine kinase MB
CMP	complete metabolic panel
CO_2	carbon dioxide
c/o	complaining of
COPD	chronic obstructive pulmonary disease
CP	chest pain
CPR	cardiopulmonary resuscitation
CSF	cerebrospinal fluid
CVA	cerebrovascular accident
DC	discharge
DIB	difficulty in breathing

DIC	disseminated intravascular coagulation
DKA	diabetic ketoacidosis
dx	diagnose
ED	emergency department
EKG	electrocardiogram
EMTALA	Emergency Treatment and Active Labor Act
ENA	Emergency Nurses Association
ENT	ear, nose, and throat
ER	emergency room
ET	endotracheal tube
ETOH	alcohol
FHT	fetal heart tones
FO	foreign object
GERD	gastroesophageal reflux disease
GI	gastrointestinal
gtts	drops
HA	headache
HCT	hematocrit
HGB	hemoglobin
HHNC	hyperosmolar, hyperglycemic nonketotic coma
HIV	human immunodeficiency virus
HOB	head of the bed
HPV	human papilloma virus
HTN	hypertension
hx	history
IBS	irritable bowel syndrome
ICP	increased cranial pressure

ICU	intensive care unit
I&D	incision and drainage
IM	intramuscular injection
INR	international normalized ratio
I&O	intake and output
IUP	intrauterine pregnancy
IV	intravenous
IVC	inferior vena cava
JVD	jugular vein distention
LFT	liver function test
LLQ	left lower quadrant
LOC	loss of consciousness
LP	lumbar puncture
LUQ	left upper quadrant
MDI	meter dose inhaler
MS	multiple sclerosis
MVI	multivitamin
NC	nasal cannula
Neb	nebulizer
NG	nasogastric
NPO	nothing by mouth
NRB	nonrebreather
NS	normal saline
NTG	nitrogylcerine
NVD	nausea/vomiting/diarrhea
O_2	oxygen
OD	overdose

OM	otitis media
OR	operating room
os	opening
PALS	pediatric advanced life support
PDA	patent ductus arteriosus
PE	pulmonary embolism
PEA	pulseless electrical activity
PEEP	positive end-expiratory pressure
PID	pelvic inflammatory disease
PIH	pregnancy-induced hypertension
PLT	platelets
PO	by mouth
PPE	personal protective equipment
pr	by rectum
PRBC	packed red blood cells
prn	as needed
PSVT	paroxysmal supraventricular tachycardia
pt	patient
PT	prothrombin time
PTT	partial thromboplastin time
PVC	premature ventricular contraction
PVD	peripheral vascular disease
q.i.d.	four times a day
q.i.w.	four times a week
resp	respiratory
RF	renal failure
RL	Ringer's Lactate
RLQ	right lower quadrant

ROM	range of motion
RSV	respiratory syncytial virus
RUQ	right upper quadrant
SC	subcutaneous
SIADH	syndrome of inappropriate antidiuretic hormone
SIDS	sudden infant death syndrome
SL	under the tongue
SOB	shortness of breath
s/s	signs and symptoms
stat	immediate
STD	sexually transmitted disease
SVT	supraventricular tachycardia
SZ	seizure
TB	tuberculosis
td	tetanus/diphtheria
TIA	transient ischemic attack
t.i.d.	three times a day
TNCC	trauma nurse core course
TSS	toxic shock syndrome
Tx	treat or treatment
UA	urinalysis
US	ultrasound
UTI	urinary tract infection
V-fib	ventricular fibrillation
VS	vital signs
VSD	ventricular septal defect
VT	ventricular tachycardia

Appendix E

Skills Check-Off Sheets

ITEM/SKILL For day 1 of orientation (no patient assignment) *Demonstration will be verbal from staff member to preceptor*	Date reviewed/ observed	Date demonstrated	Preceptor initials
Assistance notification: (supervisor, security, chaplain, DEFACS, case/risk management, ethics committee, sheriff)			
Call-in policy			
Clock-in/clock-out procedures			
Communication books and boards			
Discuss orientation needs and establish goals			
Education resources/requirements/opportunities			
Employee occurrence reports			
EMTALA guidelines			
Intercom/patient call light system			
Latex allergy protocol and procedures			
Manual time record			
Medication adverse reaction form or procedure			
Medication Occurrence Report			
Medication room			
Nursing documentation forms			
Nursing/ER policy and procedure manual			
Orient to unit/staff personnel/registration			
Orientation forms and packet			
Orientation schedule			
Patient appropriate room assignments			
Patient assignment board procedures			
Patient belongings left in department			
Patient education resources			
Patient flow in department			
Patient occurrence report			
Reference manuals			
Registration process			
Scavenger hunt			
Schedule/request form for time off/PTO			
Staffing assignments			
Storeroom supplies			
Supply room			
Telephone system			
Time and attendance policy			
Tour of department			
Videos to watch:			

ITEM/SKILL WEEK 1 Minor care/nonurgent patient assignment Review Chapters 1, 5, 14, 15	Date reviewed/ observed	Date demonstrated	Preceptor initials
Accu-chek machine and documentation			
Animal bite protocols			
Blanket warmer purpose and use			
Burn care procedures			
Care of patients assigned to (Minor Care) MCC			
Computer systems/sign up for classes			
Crash cart/Braslow cart locations			
Dermabond			
Diagnostic tests (X-ray, CT scan, MRI, VQ scan, US)			
Difficult people, working with them			
Discharge procedures and instructions			
Ear irrigation/Morgan eye lens			
Evaluation form, reassess goals weekly			
Eye exams supplies: Wood's lamp, eye kit, slit lamp			
Immobilization and splinting techniques (Ortho-Glass)			
Incision and drainage procedures			
Instrument recycling (disposable/nondisposable)			
Joint commission information			
Language translation methods (verbal/written)			
Material safety data sheets (MSDS)			
Minor care policies and procedures			
Medication administration policies and procedures			
Pain assessment and documentation			
Pain management policy/procedures			
Positioning and securing of pediatric patient (papoose)			
Rapid Strep screen collection procedure			
Respiratory aerosol nebulizer treatment			
Supplies for MCC nonurgent			
Suture/staple removal procedure			
Suture/wound care supplies, protocols, techniques			
Tetanus prophylaxis			
Treatment of minors in the ED			
Urine collection procedures			
Use/purpose of soiled utility room			
Use/purpose/flow of patients in minor care department			
Visual acuity (adult or pediatric)			
Worker's compensation drug screening			

ITEM/SKILL WEEKS 2–4 Nonurgent patient and pelvic room assignment Review Chapters 6, 7, 8, 9, 13	Date reviewed/ observed	Date demonstrated	Preceptor initials
Abuse/neglect evaluation			
AMA (patient leaving against medical advice) procedures			
Assessments: primary, secondary, focused			
BEAR hugger uses/purposes			
Blood work interpretation			
Care of priority three or nonurgent patients			
C-spine immobilization and removal techniques			
Documentation of assessment/treatment/medication			
Doppler: vessel and obstetric uses			
EMS radio and H.E.A.R. system radio			
Evaluation form, reassess goals weekly			
Fetal Heart monitoring in ED			
Finger Traps			
Foley catheter removal			
Foley catheterization, urine meter			
GYN exam/specimens and products of conception			
Head lamp			
IV insertion (INT) procedures			
IV infusion pumps			
Left without treatment procedures			
Methotrexate for ectopic pregnancy			
Miscarriage (complete/incomplete) referrals			
Morgan eye lens/eye irrigation techniques			
Nonurgent patient acuity			
Nosebleed procedures and equipment			
Pain assessment and documentation			
Patient teaching documentation			
Pelvic stretchers			
Pelvic supplies			
Phlebotomy check-off, venipunctures Lab and INT			
Portable monitor systems			
Precipitous delivery procedures and supplies			
Rape/sexual assault examination protocol			
Rapid flu specimen collection			
RhoGAM/blood product administration			
(RSV)Respiratory syncytial virus specimen collection			
Stool specimen collection			
Urinary catheterization procedures, Quik cath (8fr, 5fr)			
Urology cart/supplies			
Use/purpose/flow in the nonurgent rooms			
Vital sign monitoring of nonurgent patients			

ITEM/SKILL WEEKS 5–8 Urgent patient assignment Review Chapters 2, 10, 11, 16, 17	Date reviewed/ observed	Date demonstrated	Preceptor initials
1013/2013 forms			
12-lead ECG check-off and interpretation			
Acute allergic reaction (anaphylaxis)			
Admission procedure			
Advanced directives and DNR status			
Airway open/maintain: nontrauma and trauma			
Airway/breathing supplies and usage in ED			
Anesthesia consent			
Arterial blood gas interpretation			
Bag valve mask: adult, pediatric, neonatal			
Blood/blood products administration and forms			
Central port access (gripper/Huber needle)			
Central vein access kit and procedures			
Crash cart, Braslow cart			
Endotracheal intubation and rapid-sequence intubation			
Evaluation form, reassess goals weekly			
Gastric lavage/Lavacuator tube, NG tube (oral/nasal)			
GI bleed procedures			
Hare traction splint			
Hemoccult/stool/gastric specimen collection			
Holding of admitted patients			
Lumbar puncture tray, procedure/patient position			
Mental health patient care			
Monitoring system: central, bedside, portable			
Neonate patient care			
Neutropenia policy and procedures			
OR admission and preoperative checklist			
Patient transfer procedure and transfer			
Pediatric care and reference manuals			
Peritoneal lavage			
Purpose/use/flow of urgent room assignments			
Respiratory care check-off			
Seclusion/restraint policy			
Secondary assessments and reassessments			
Security policy regarding mental health patients			
Sedation and analgesia policy and procedures/forms			
Sputum specimen collection procedures			
Surgical consent			
Tuberculosis suspected patient care			
Urgent patient acuity			
Urgent patient supplies			
Ventilator troubleshooting and patient care			

ITEM/SKILL WEEKS 9–12 Priority 1 emergent patient and triage assignment Review Chapters 3, 4, 12, 18, 19	Date reviewed/ observed	Date demonstrated	Preceptor initials
ACLS and PALS protocols			
Biphasic/monophasic defibrillator			
Cardiac arrhythmias			
Chest tube equipment/procedures: hemo/pneumothorax			
Code blue form and code blue critique form			
Code blue procedure in the ED			
Code blue procedures out of the ED			
Crash cart			
Cricothyrotomy kit and procedure			
Death in the department/physician pronouncements			
Deceased patient data form			
Decontamination equipment			
Defibrillator/pacer procedures			
Disaster plan			
Emergency medications and resource manual			
Emergent acuity patients			
Emergent patient supplies			
ER nurse's role in code blue			
Evaluation form and revise goals weekly			
Heimlich valve			
Infusion protocols (cardiac/emergency infusions)			
Level 1 rapid infuser/fluid warming equipment/supplies			
MAST (Military Anti-Shock Trousers)			
Multiple trauma patient care			
Needle decompression			
Neurological assessment/documentation			
Patient priority setting			
Pericardiocentesis tray			
Pervenous temporary pacemaker			
Poison control notification/documentation			
Pregnant trauma patient care			
Seizure precautions and patient care			
Tackle boxes for TPA, allergy, transport, TNKase, RSI			
TPA/TNKase policies/procedures: Acute MI, stroke			
Tracheostomy tray and procedure			
Transcutaneous pacemaker procedure			
Transport defibrillator procedures			
Transport of critical patient			
Triage guidelines/protocols (disaster and non-disaster)			
Use/purpose/flow priority 1 or trauma rooms			
Complete post orientation evaluation form assessment of the clinical orientation process, review goals, and assess need for orientation extension			

References

Centers for Disease Control and Prevention. (2009). *Bioterrorism & chemical emergencies.* Retrieved June 17, 2009, from http://www.bt.cdc.gov/

Dallas, C. E., Coule, P. L., James, J. J., Lillibridge, S., Pepe, P. E., Schwartz, R. B., et al. (Eds.). (2004). *Basic disaster life support provider manual version 2.5.* Chicago: American Medical Association.

Emergency Nurses Association. (2001, Revised printing 2004). *CEN review manual* (3rd ed.). Dubuque, IA: Kendal Hunt.

Emergency Nurses Association. (2007). *Emergency nursing core curriculum* (6th ed.). Philadelphia: Saunders.

Emergency Nurses Association. (2007). *Trauma nurse core course: Provider manual* (6th ed.). Des Plaines, IL: Author.

Field, J. M., Hazinski, M. F., & Gilmor, D. (Eds.). (2005). *Handbook of emergency cardiovascular care.* Salem, MA: American Heart Association.

Gasparis Vonfrolio, L. (1999). *The one and only CEN review course.* Staten Island, NY: Education Enterprises.

Goldstein, M. (Dec. 2008). Carbon monoxide poisoning. *Journal of Emergency Nursing, 34*(6), 538–541.

Hacker, N., Gambone, J. C., & Moore, J. G. (2004). *Essentials of obstetrics and gynecology* (4th ed.). Philadelphia: Elsevier Health Sciences.

Hamilton, R. (2009). *Tarascon pocket pharmacopoeia.* Sudbury, MA: Jones & Bartlett.

Hanlon, D., & Duriseti, R. (May-June, 2001). Current concepts in the management of the pregnant trauma patient. *Trauma Reports,* 2(3), 1–10.

Hohenhaus, S. M. (2008). In the news and in our practice: Pediatric emergencies. *ENA Connection, 32*(7), 1.

Kenneth, S. S. (2006). *Anatomy and physiology: The unity of form and function* (4th ed.). New York: McGraw-Hill.

Knoop, K. J., Stack, L. B., & Storrow, A. B. (Eds.). (2002). *Atlas of emergency medicine* (2nd ed.). New York: McGraw-Hill.

Kolecki, P., & Menckhoff, C. R. (2008). *Shock, Hypovolemic.* Retrieved October 10, 2008, from http://www.emedicine.com/ped/topic118.htm

Mayo Clinic. (2008). *Diseases and conditions.* Retrieved September 10, 2008, from http://www.mayoclinic.com/

Newerry, L. (Ed.). (2002). *Sheehy's emergency nursing principles and practice* (5th ed.). St Louis: Mosby-Year Book.

Oman, K., & Kozoll-McLain, J. (Eds.). (2006). *Emergency nursing secrets* (2nd ed.). Philadelphia: Elsevier Health Sciences.

Pagana, K.D., & Pagana, J.T. (2005). *Mosby's manual of diagnostic and laboratory tests* (3rd ed.). Philadelphia: Elsevier Health Sciences.

Rothrock, G. S. (2005). *Tarascon adult emergency pocketbook.* Winter Park, FL: Mako Publishing.

Schilling McCann, J. A. (2004). *Lippincott's Q & A certification review emergency nursing.* Philadelphia: Lippincott Williams & Wilkins.

Skidmore-Roth, L. (2009). *Mosby's nursing drug reference.* St. Louis: Mosby.

Tintinalli, J. E., Kelen, G. D., & Stapczynski, J. S. (Eds.). (2003). *Emergency medicine: A comprehensive study guide* (6th ed.). New York: McGraw-Hill.

Videbeck, S.L. (2007). *Psychiatric mental health nursing.* Philadelphia: Lippincott.

Wong, D. L. (1999). *Whaley & Wong's nursing care of infants and children* (6th ed.). St. Louis: Mosby.

Index

Other FAST FACTS Books

Fast Facts for the NEW NURSE PRACTITIONER*: What You Really Need to Know in a Nutshell,* Aktan

Fast Facts for the ER NURSE*: Emergency Room Orientation in a Nutshell,* Buettner

Fast Facts for the CLINICAL NURSE MANAGER*: Managing a Changing Workplace in a Nutshell,* Fry

Fast Facts for EVIDENCE-BASED PRACTICE*: Implementing EBP in a Nutshell,* Godshall

Fast Facts for the TRAVEL NURSE*: Travel Nursing in Nutshell,* Landrum

Fast Facts for the MEDICAL OFFICE NURSE*: What You Really Need to Know in a Nutshell,* Richmeier

Fast Facts for CAREER SUCCESS IN NURSING*: Making the Most of Mentoring in a Nutshell,* Vance

Fast Facts for the CLINICAL NURSING INSTRUCTOR*: Clinical Teaching in Nutshell,* Zabat Kan, Stabler-Haas

Forthcoming

Fast Facts for the FAITH COMMUNITY NURSE*: Implementing FCN/Parish Nursing in a Nutshell,* Hickman

Fast Facts for the CARDIAC SURGERY NURSE*: Everything You Need to Know in a Nutshell,* Hodge

Fast Facts for the WOUND CARE NURSE*: Practical Wound Management in a Nutshell,* Kifer

Fast Facts for the CRITICAL CARE NURSE*: Critical Care Nursing in a Nutshell,* Landrum

Fast Facts for the SCHOOL NURSE*: School Nursing in a Nutshell,* Loschiavo

Fast Facts for the PSYCHIATRIC NURSE*: Psychiatric Mental Health Nursing in a Nutshell,* Masters

Fast Facts for DEMENTIA CARE*: What Nurses Need to Know in a Nutshell,* Miller

Fast Facts about the GYNECOLOGICAL EXAM *for* NURSE PRACTITIONERS*: Conducting the GYN Exam in a Nutshell,* Secor

Fast Facts about DEVELOPING *a* NURSING ACADEMIC PORTFOLIO*: What to Include in a Nutshell,* Wittmann-Price

Fast Facts for the CLASSROOM NURSING INSTRUCTOR*: Classroom Teaching in a Nutshell,* Yoder-Wise, Kowalski